Secret Doctors

Secret Doctors

ETHNOMEDICINE OF AFRICAN AMERICANS

Wonda L. Fontenot

Bergin & Garvey
WESTPORT, CONNECTICUT · LONDON

Library of Congress Cataloging-in-Publication Data

Fontenot, Wonda L.
   Secret doctors : ethnomedicine of African Americans / Wonda L.
Fontenot.
       p.   cm.
   Pref. and acknowledgements
   Includes bibliographical references and index.
   ISBN 0–89789–354–9 (alk. paper)
   1. Traditional medicine—Louisiana.   2. Afro-Americans—Louisiana—
Medicine.   3. Afro-Americans—Louisiana—Religion.   4. Afro-
Americans—Louisiana—Rites and ceremonies.   5. Louisiana—Social
life and customs.   I. Title.
GR110.L5F47   1994
615.8'82'08996073—dc20   93–40560

British Library Cataloguing in Publication Data is available.

Library of Congress Catalog Card Number: 93–40560
ISBN: 0–89789–354–9

First published in 1994

Bergin & Garvey, 88 Post Road West, Westport, CT 06881
An imprint of Greenwood Publishing Group, Inc.

Printed in the United States of America

The paper used in this book complies with the
Permanent Paper Standard issued by the National
Information Standards Organization (Z39.48–1984).

10 9 8 7 6 5 4 3 2 1

Copyright Acknowledgment

An earlier version of Chapter 4 appeared in Wonda Lee Fontenot, "Madame Neau:
The Practice of Ethno-Psychiatry in Rural Louisiana," in Barbara Bair and Susan E.
Cayleff, eds., *Wings of Gauze: Women of Color and the Experience of Health and
Illness* (Detroit: Wayne State University Press, 1993). Copyright © 1993 by Wayne
State University Press. Reprinted with permission.

To the memory of my mother
Emma Lou Jack-Fontenot
(1927–1983)

and to my nieces and nephews
Rhonda, Greg, Twaski, Aleadra, Tara, Donald, Jr., Eric, Kaia,
Rachel Emma, and Kisache.

Contents

Maps and Figures

Preface

This book evolved out of immense love, pride, and respect for the African-American secret doctoring tradition. The process of achieving a terminal degree led to the initial stages of gathering data, later to become the basis for the book you now hold. I hoped this data would clarify many misconceptions about the origins and justification of African-American medical beliefs and practices. I felt compelled, having endured this medical tradition, to speak out regarding the integrity of a tradition that was indeed, at one time, the only source of medicine available to the African-American masses. My compulsion was strengthened as I encountered literature, both popular and scholarly, that often ill defined or excluded factual data that would enhance one's understanding not only of contemporary beliefs associated with illness, but also clarify how Afrocentric religious dogma governs behavior associated with beliefs and practices related to illness, health, and socialization.

Descriptives such as bizarre, exotic, etc., were foreign to me and contradictory to the experience I had growing up in rural Louisiana. What became profoundly important was to offer explanations that demonstrate that there is nothing extraordinarily different about African-American ethnomedicine from that of other folk medicine belief systems. To fully understand the historical and social conditions that shape the African-American medical experience, a holistic approach must be taken. It is not an isolated phenomenon, but rather a fraction of the whole.

The process that led to the writing of this book was no ordinary experience. It was joyful, cathartic, and sometimes painful, but I always had an unyielding passion to tell this story. It was the beginning of my discovery of the broader history of people of African descent. Let me be clear I was familiar with the history of people of African descent, but from an oral tradition—family narratives as told by my father, mother, grandfather, and other ancestors. But it was those analytical probing truths that were foreign to me, such as the scientific rationale for why people believe in spirits, reasons for syncopation in music, etc., common to the American African as it was to the Haitian, the West African, and others of the African diaspora.

It was with my mother that my affinity for secret doctoring was realized. This experience, in addition to other religious and social events too enormous to cite here, led to my reading *Island Possessed* by Katherine Dunham. Thus began my first exploration of kinship links between Haiti and Louisiana and their many shared cultural values. My many visits to Haiti eventually led me to West Africa; and my visionary journey to Liberia, Ghana, and Nigeria led me back home to Louisiana. Thus the circle was created but not completed. Over a period of three and one half years, I was completely absorbed in why people got sick, how they got well, and what they believed caused their maladies. I wanted to hear from believers themselves, and it seemed as though no scholarship offered me any complete explanation. I had no idea what it was I was hoping to find, because initially I thought the answers were to be found in Haiti or West Africa. However, the more I asked questions and conducted research, the more questions surfaced in relation to the African-American ethnomedicine tradition. Perhaps it took my travels abroad to legitimize my growing and overwhelming concern and interest in my own more immediate heritage—the African American ethnomedicine experience in rural Louisiana in specific and in the United States in general—an interest and concern which led to this document that I believe is a guidepost of sorts—a start—a document which invites individuals to begin to look at a people's beliefs and customs through culturally-sensitive eyes.

The magnitude of the task before me was one that I accepted graciously. I realized that current literature was not enough, and that my nieces and nephews, and other children like them, needed to understand their heritage from an insider's point of view. I saw the need to document and provide historically accurate data on a tradition that is slowly becoming extinct. I realized that outsiders also needed another reference point or source from which they could draw, expand, and begin to examine.

The result is an ethnohistorical study of the medical tradition of African Americans. The study posits that this medical (secret doctoring) tradition is an expression of their West African heritage. This study seeks to determine what role regional and cultural continuity has in the traditional thoughts and ideas of the people as revealed in their present day folk medical system.

The study also looks at selected African-American folk medical traditions retained and what determined their retention. Additionally, because the issue of cultural mixing is important to this region, another concern addressed in the book is the influence of the triad culture (Native American, European, and African) on the evolution of this medical system. What developed from this triad culture was medico-religious practices and beliefs that incorporated West and Central African theology, Christian elements, and were influenced by Native American traditions.

The study concludes that this is a viable medical system based on oral tradition, trust, and common cultural values and beliefs about illness and its causes. It is characterized by both Baptists and Catholics whose religious practices are based simultaneously on orthodox religious doctrines and non-orthodox religious healing customs. Thus, prayer, faith, and the power of the spirit of God embodied within a material object became the key Christian elements for healing rituals of African Americans in rural French Louisiana.

Acknowledgments

Many persons contributed in some way or another to make this study possible. I am grateful to Secret Doctors and persons in St. Landry, Evangeline, and Acadia Parishes who helped me further my research by offering suggestions, contacts, support, and entrusting me with such valuable and cherished information so that I might accurately document this African-American medical tradition.

Special thanks to Professors William Simmons, Barbara Christian, and James Deetz for their guidance during the initial writing of this book. Professor Simmons motivated my triadic approach to this research. He was always genuinely interested in the material and was also prompt and particularly motivating during the times of my field research. Professor Deetz enthusiastically encouraged my material culture approach, and Professor Christian influenced originality in my ethnographic writing. She was my cheerleader. Sheila Walker provided excellent content comments which helped shape the focus. Yvonne Daniel was a "big sister" through it all and was there for me when I needed her emotionally, spiritually, and academically. Also professors William Shack, Margaret Wilkerson, and Roy Thomas were equally supportive.

It is impossible to name all my relatives, friends, and colleagues who helped. However special thanks to my aunts Bert, Earline, Leona, Ruby, Gladys, and Elmae, and cousin Denise. They all in some way lifted me spiritually when I needed it, and they were firm when I vacillated. Marcella Ford, Ella Bogan, Roland Foulkes, and my good friends Linda Miller, Curtis Taylor, Carolyn Lee, Donna Hephinger, Phillis Walker, Malonga Casquelourd, and my cohorts in Malonga's congolese dance class, Leona, Constance, Arnita, and Cherise, were also encouraging.

I am also indebted to my husband, father, sisters, and brother. They stood by me and helped make much of my work possible. Daddy, who has always been concerned, provided the foundation—he was our family griot (an oral historian in the West African tradition). My sisters Mable and Linda, and my brother Hayward, Jr., all offered sibling blessings. The greatest supporter and source of my inspiration is my husband, Wilken Jones, Jr. It was his love and unwavering belief in my mission that carried me over. I also thank Almighty God for giving me strength and determination.

Introduction

Louisiana has a unique history. It is a state that has an exotic cultural tradition with strong remnants of French, West African, and Native American cultures. Louisiana was once a French and Spanish colony, late 1600s–1762 and 1762–1802 respectively, before it became the property of the United States of America. The U.S. acquisition came in 1803. The largest and most culturally rich early settlements in Louisiana were and remain New Orleans and French-speaking rural southwest Louisiana. A strong surviving tradition in rural Louisiana is the African-American religious-based medical tradition, whose practitioners are known as "Secret Doctors" or "Treaters." This folk medicine tradition has its origin in West Africa.

In southwest Louisiana issues of ethnicity are also prevalent and significant. Racial/ethnic labels, such as African Americans, Native Americans, White, Black, Free Person of Color, Black Indians, Creole, Mulatto, Colored, Cajuns, etc., are common in the history of Louisiana. Historically, these racial/ethnic labels once determined a person's social status, as well as their freedom to go and come as they chose. Today some of these racial/ethnic identifications are not as obvious; but an ethnic identity crisis presently remains in southwest Louisiana. Locals, and outsiders, struggle to define or clarify what is African American or Creole.[1] Dominguez (1986) and Cobb and Cobb (1977) are scholars who have examined the issue of race and ethnicity in Louisiana.

Mixed blood heritage is a very real part of this African-American society. The aftermath of intermarriage and intermingling between African Americans, Native Americans, and French and Spanish Europeans, are topics that have received some attention from historians and cultural studies' scholars—but

Map I.1
French Mother Tongue: U.S.-Born Black Population (Southern Louisiana, 1970)

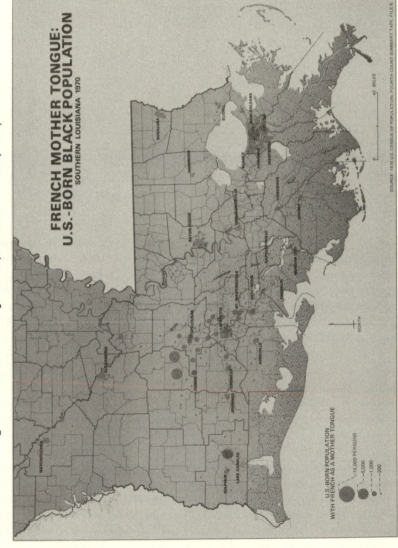

Source: Produced by James P. Allen and the Cartography Lab, Department of Geography, California State University, Northridge.

not nearly enough. African and American Indian mixing particularly, is an issue that needs more exploration, especially as it relates to the ethnic identity and the cultural traditions of African Americans in the southeastern United States.

Many Louisiana persons proudly say that they can speak French, Creole, or Creole French, as it is variously called by contemporaries. Persons are also proud of their French and Spanish heritages, and those persons who are descendants of old French families (original settlers) are held in high esteem. The French speaking African Americans are no exception; they too, are proud of their French and Spanish as well as African heritage.

Those who claim it are equally proud of their Native American ancestry. Rarely do you hear a genealogy recited without the reciter boasting about a French or Spanish ancestor, usually French. Some openly admit their Native American heritage and point to photos that grace their walls showing off their mixed blood Native American kinfolks. Others, hesitant, bring out old dusty photos of a parent or grandparent that was "Indian."

The extent to which I explore the phenomenon of cultural and racial mixing between African Americans and Native Americans is limited to the oral history accounts of mixed heritage individuals in this study. This is a very complicated and broad topic, and it is much too important to go unnoticed. Native American and African American intermixing is a subject that has, more often than not, gone unacknowledged although it has been addressed by some scholars (Crowe 1975; Hudson 1975; Katz 1986; Kniffen 1987; Potter 1932; Simmons 1986; Sturtevant 1963; Swanton 1946; Wright 1981).

My examination of racial mixing and intermingling between African Americans and early Europeans is, in some ways, an in-depth approach. This is an area that has been adequately documented, and literature about this mixed blood group crosses many disciplines, perhaps because this mixed blood heritage has had the most profound effect on African American people, both inter- and intraculturally.[2] It created class distinctions, skin color prejudices, and a whole array of psychological and social concerns and upheavals—many that have been addressed, and many that have not. A widely documented subject, literary sources cite the many toils and burdens of being "neither black nor white" in early Louisiana. An awkward position, but a position that was nonetheless responsible for creating the present class and color structure in Louisiana.

For the most part there is nothing unusual about these Louisiana people of African descent. They are just ordinary rural people. Most of them are farmers or descendants of farmers. What sets them apart from the rest of the world—outside Louisiana—is that most of them were Franco Africans before they became Americans.

Focus on a specific community makes for a manageable research project with limited possibilities for errors. Many errors of interpretation were committed by previous researchers who tended to view rural southern African

Americans as having the same customs. Although there are many cultural similarities among African Americans, there are many differences. Such studies failed to consider the multiple causes for African-American cultural dissimilarities, related to such factors as demographics, regional differences, cultural heritage, political structure, and language.

This study therefore focuses specifically on the ethnographic treatment of one African-American community in rural French Louisiana; however, the conceptual issues raised relates to the collective historical conditions of African Americans in the rural South. I especially seek to find out what role cultural continuity has in the thoughts and ideas of the people, as revealed today in their folk medical system where Africanisms still survive. Bascom 1972, Bastide 1971, Cole 1985, Davis 1958, Herskovits 1969, Levine 1977, Mintz and Price 1976, and Walker 1980 are a few of the scholars who argue in favor of surviving Africanisms. Studies by Deetz 1977, Edwards 1976–1980, Holloway (1990), Thompson 1984, and Vlach 1978, are important in studying surviving Africanisms from a material culture perspective.

Research done on African-American traditional medicine as a medical system is limited. Additionally, it is rare that African-American medical traditions have been documented, or thought worthy of scientific investigation as a "medical system," having rational, logical order and meaning (Hill 1976). Often these studies fail to analyze the medical tradition as a means to better understand cultural beliefs, behavior, and attitudes associated with the causes and cures for illnesses among African Americans.

The review of the literature reveals that studies done on African-American folk medicine by outsiders are often not totally accurate and in some cases (for example, Louisiana), they are practically nonexistent. Some important studies are dated. During the early twentieth century, African Americans were called Colored or Negro, and Native Americans, like African Americans, were not yet socially integrated into mainstream America. Much of the scholarship of those times reflects the Eurocentric attitudes toward People of Color.

Traditional medicine in rural Louisiana, the focus of this study, shares conceptual similarities cross-culturally, especially as it relates to practices and beliefs operating alongside religion and magic. Scholars whose theoretical considerations guided my conceptual developments regarding medicine and magical practices are: Bell 1980; Budge 1930; Frazer 1958; Hand 1964, 1980; Haskins 1974; Honko 1962–63; Hyatt 1973; Jackson 1980; Laguerre 1987; Nassau 1904; Rivers 1924; Roheim 1930; Snow 1977a, 1977b, 1986; and Tylor 1920.

Studies done specifically on African-American traditional medical beliefs and practices in Louisiana are also limited (Roberts 1927; Tallant 1967; Webb 1971). From an African-American native's point of view, the scholarship is nonexistent for Louisiana. Hurston (1935), an African American but a non-native, did make some observations on traditional medical beliefs and practices in Louisiana.

Religion is very much a part of the healing tradition of these African-American folk doctors. Christian prayers and unorthodox religious customs, such as the use of amulets, play a key role in Secret Doctors healing rituals. Some theologians and historians who have examined the African American religious experience and/or the folk customs associated with religious worship style are: Boles 1943; Carter 1976; Cone 1984; Frazier 1966; Hurston 1983; Jones-Jackson 1987; Joyner 1984; Long 1986; Mitchell 1975; Mitchell 1986; Raboteau 1980; Seale and Seale 1942; Sobel 1979; Stampp 1956; and Washington 1964.

Folk medicine[3] is a topic of particular concern for me, because of my concern with mainstream medicine's lack of cultural awareness of the health beliefs of African Americans, the quality of health care for Blacks, and inadequate and often ineffective health care delivery systems in rural areas. In addition, issues like traditional values and religion as they relate to medicine are equally important. I selected rural Louisiana for a regional focus because of the survival of indigenous cultural traits and because of my familiarity, as a native, with the region on a geographic as well as a cultural basis.[4]

Being no stranger to this community, I was able to enter with a certain amount of ease. The secret doctors trusted me because of who I was—one of them. As I began to broaden my intellectual base via my academic pursuits, I became curious about the conceptual issues related to traditional medicine among rural African-American populations. I wanted to know why people were continuously utilizing dual medical systems (mainstream and traditional). What was it in one that maybe didn't work in the other medical system? Did this dual system of medicine operate in other parts of the United States or other parts of rural Louisiana? Was it operating among other ethnic groups? As I read about similar practices, I then began to question why African-American medical practices were viewed in such bad taste in some scholarship, such as Webb's (1971) study. While on the other hand treatment of data related to traditional medical practices and beliefs of Latin Americans and Chinese Americans, for example, warranted a different kind of analysis—one which made attempts to respect cultural diversity and excite the intellect. I was particularly concerned about the way outsiders analyzed the medical tradition of African Americans and whether these early scholars were misguided as outsiders. What did it mean to secret doctors who lived at a certain point in time, in a certain space as African Americans with traditional beliefs and values, and what did it mean for those before them? What is it they practice and how? Why do they maintain traditional medical practices and who are their patients?

I believe that there is a common religious sentiment among all people of the African diaspora; hence I believe that there are no sharp discontinuities between African Americans in other parts of the United States and those in Louisiana, especially in rural areas. All African people of the New World share

African heritage, and all share a common experience of enslavement. What differentiates one African of the Americas from another is a difference in cultural orientation. For example, a key period in the history of African Americans in Louisiana was the colonial period. The years prior to 1803 marked the emergence of the present indigenous bilingual African-American community. During this period extensive migration occurred between Louisiana and Haiti, causing a multifaceted society to develop. African, Caribbean, Native American, French European, and White American elements mixed (Dunbar-Nelson 1916, 1917; Berlin 1976; Fiehrer 1979).

Louisiana was very much part of the Caribbean cultural area until 1803; the year when it was bought by the United States. It was considered a sister island to Haiti. Haitian culture, as a result, played an extremely important role in helping to shape the early African-American folklife of Louisiana. This was evident in certain early dance forms, religion, material culture, architectural design, foodways, and similarities in Creole language (Vlach 1978; Edwards 1980; Emery 1988).

Migration, colonization, and a system of religious and slave laws created what I have termed a "triad" culture consisting of African, Native American, and European. This socio-cultural combination was distinctive to the United States and particularly to Louisiana. One of the most astonishing developments from this triadic culture was the evolution of religious practices that utilized both African and Christian elements and ideologies to form a syncretic belief system. It was in the eighteenth century that present day Louisiana African-American religious practices with their psychocultural intricacies originated.

It was during my travels to Haiti and West Africa that I first observed cross-cultural similarities between Haiti, West Africa, and African Americans in rural Louisiana. More importantly, it was at this time in my life that I realized that African-American culture in rural Louisiana was in need of studying and recording from an insider's perspective. So I returned home to Louisiana, and I began researching traditional medical beliefs and practices. My research travels and studies also confirmed that people of the African diaspora expressed differences and similarities in their beliefs and practices associated with traditional medicine.

Scholars whose works document traditional medicine in cultures of the African diaspora and who I found important are: Hill 1976; Mitchell 1978; Murphree 1976; and West 1975. I found these works especially insightful because I was interested in finding out what it was about the Louisiana African-Americans' traditional cultural experiences that made them different or similar to these African American and African cultures. In addition I was interested in finding out how much, or what aspects, of this practice was credited by these secret doctors to their African heritage.

French values, the Codes Noir (slave laws), and racial mixtures, have had a lasting influence on Louisiana society. In spite of profound experiences

(Christian conversion, enslavement, and ethnic and cultural mixing), this indigenous medical system among African Americans in rural Louisiana survives.

RESEARCH METHODS

Because I was especially interested in people's own life experiences as secret doctors, I collected oral history accounts from secret doctors as the primary means of gathering data for this study. Participation in and observation of healing rituals added additional insight into this ethnomedical tradition. I also conducted interviews, using open- and closed-ended questions. The interviews were with secret doctors, patients, community leaders, and members. In addition data was collected utilizing ethnobotany and archival methods.

Initially thirty-three secret doctors were identified, and a preliminary interview was conducted with twenty-three of them. From these twenty-three, ten secret doctors were selected for in-depth study because aspects of their folk medical knowledge, or technique, contributed to the cohesiveness of this study. The secret doctors represent a cross-section of persons with African descent, varying in age, sex, religious denomination, and social status.

Four of the secret doctors are females who range in age from thirty-six to eighty-six. I chose two of the women because of their experience, not only as secret doctors, but also as midwives. I chose another woman because of her mixed heritage (Native American and African American), and because her methods of treatment are influenced by modernization. The other woman was chosen because of her unique talent as an ethnopsychiatrist.

The six male secret doctors range in age from sixty-three to eighty-eight. All of the men selected use herb plants in treating practices. I selected one because of his mixed heritage (Native American and African American) and knowledge of medicinal herbs, and another also because of his extensive knowledge of native medicinal herbs. I selected two others because of their use of unusual ritual artifacts—amulets. I chose the fifth secret doctor because of his use of amulets and his strong recollection of historical facts; and the sixth male secret doctor was selected because he used an altar in his treating rituals.

ORGANIZATION OF CHAPTERS

Three major components are central to this research project. They are: (1) the socio-cultural history of the area as well as the cultural groups in the region (Chapters 1 and 2); (2) the history, development, and contemporary aspects of folk medicine as it relates to race and gender, especially that of African Americans in general and particularly in rural Louisiana (Chapters 3, 4, and 5); (3) the elements which dominate African-American treating rituals—religion and ritual artifacts (the belief in the supernatural and the use of prayer, amulets, and medicinal plants). These factors reveal the strongest African continuities (Chapters 6, 7, and 8).

Chapter 1 gives a historical account of the setting of this research. It focuses on the social history and organization of Louisiana from the late 1600s to 1803, when Louisiana was sold by the French to the United States of America. In describing the period 1690–1719, I provide an overview of the life of existing Native Americans to the time of the arrival of the French to Louisiana, focusing on the southwest region and the beginning of development of Louisiana as a state. In the period covering 1720 to 1750, I give an account of the beginning of importation of Africans to Louisiana and to the southwest area and some early observations regarding plantation systems, customs, and social status of the enslaved African in the South and in Louisiana during the plantation era.

Therefore, Chapter 1 concerns the history of African Americans in Louisiana, as well as preliminary observations of other cultural groups of the area and their ethnic history. The chapter concludes with a look at the contemporary socio-economic situation of Louisiana in general and rural southwest Louisiana in particular, especially as it relates to African Americans.

Chapter 2 is concerned with the history of the folk medicine tradition of African Americans. It begins with an introduction to West African folk medicine tradition and ritual practices. Folk medicine as it existed in the South, and Louisiana in general, and particularly as it relates to the enslaved and freed African, during the plantation and post emancipation era, is discussed. Also of importance in this chapter is a discussion as to how the present medical tradition of African Americans has been historically defined—how it developed, what function it served, and how it has been maintained, although modified, despite the conditions of slavery.

In Chapter 3 I summarize the oral history accounts of African-Americans' folk medicine in rural Louisiana, as remembered and told by surviving secret doctors. Some of these secret doctors have origins in other parts of the South and have foreparents who were secret doctors.

This folk medicine tradition represents an oral form of doctrine; thus the ethnographic data is presented in the secret doctors' own voices. This narrative form introduces the reader to these secret doctors, their language and lifestyles, in a very intimate way. The chapter concludes with an analysis of what it means to be a secret doctor and the common patterns of practices between them.

Chapter 4 is concerned with the specifics of mental illness and its causes and treatment practices. I examine a particular mind reader/ethnopsychiatrist's (the equivalent of a psychoanalyst) life history as a means of exploring the divining elements of this African based tradition.

My approach in Chapter 5 is historical and ethnographic. It is especially concerned with the role of African-American women as ritual specialists, as health care providers, and as recipients of health care. It is also particularly concerned with the perceptions of illness and health as defined by African-American women, and the role they played in traditional medicine, as well as their role in shaping, or as victims, of the mainstream medical system, in light of their own experiences and that of other women in general. This is an important chapter in that literature about African-American rural women is practically nonexistent.

In Chapter 6 I examine prayer (types, functions, structure) and supernatural beliefs which I view as essential to the healing ritual. There are three types of prayers defined—the secret prayer, the call and response, and the prayer proverb. The prayers themselves are not secret but what prayer is said when, and for what illness, is considered secret. The prayer tradition of African Americans is explained to show the relationship between healing ritual prayers and that of the prayers said in prayer meetings of Protestant congregations. Prayer as a means to communicate with supernatural beings, and summon— in this case God and the Holy Spirit—is a correlation with the function of prayer as commonly practiced by ritual specialists of the African diaspora. Prayer as all encompassing power is not a foreign element to persons of African descent. The chapter ends by relating the importance of prayer in healing to the pious nature of the secret doctors.

In Chapter 7 I focus on ritual artifacts and their cultural link to West Africa, particularly that of the Congo. This chapter is specifically concerned with how this aspect—animist beliefs—of the medical tradition exhibits the strongest concept of surviving Africanism. Nine ritual artifacts (amulets) are identified, along with their function. In this chapter the importance of belief in spiritual beings having life becomes very clear. Also, the struggle for a balance between good and evil is prevalent. This struggle is not uncommon, as it exists in other genres of African-American culture.

Chapter 8 documents the medical ethnobotany tradition in this African-American milieu. This chapter validates another area of this medical tradition that has been given very little attention as an African-American knowledge base. This ethnobotany chapter, or knowledge of medicinal plants, is also crucial because it reinforces the notion of early social intermingling between Africans and Indians. Many secret doctors credit their knowledge of plants to a Native American ancestor. Thirty-three medicinal plants are identified along with discussion on how they are gathered, prepared, and used.

Many of the traditional ways of these African Americans have gone undocumented. Like many oral traditions where the written word does not dominate, part of that history is lost when certain members who are the carriers of the oral history die. Three of the secret doctors died during my research stay in Louisiana. We also find gaps in African-American history as significant events, knowledge, etc., are not recorded or are ill recorded.

I intend with this study to record this oral tradition, to reveal the complexities of the African-American medical system, to encourage cultural sensitivity among mainstream medicine practitioners, by putting forth Afrocentric cultural beliefs about health, illness, and its causes, and to challenge existing scholarship on this subject by offering an insider's point of view.

NOTES

1. There are several good local sources that address this issue and attempt to define how persons of mixed heritage in Louisiana define their ethnicity. Two such sources are: "Creole Controversy," a documentary by Peggy Scott Laborde, New Orleans, La: WYES, October 1989; and "Identity Crisis," *Lafayette* (Louisiana) *Times of Acadiana*, July 26, 1989.

2. Langston Hughes, *Mulatto* in *Five Plays by Langston Hughes*, Ed. Webster Smalley (Bloomington: Indiana University Press, 1969).

3. Ethnomedicine, treating, traditional medicine, and folk medicine are corresponding terms. Folk doctor, secret doctor, traditional practitioner, and treaters are also equivalents. However, terms used in the community are not the terms used in anthropology. For the purpose of clarity, I will use them interchangeably.

4. This is an exploratory ethnography, and it does not claim to be a conclusive study.

Secret Doctors

1

Historic and Contemporary
Opelousas Territory

HISTORIC COMMUNITY

In my research for this chapter, I collected baseline data about the original
Opelousas Territory (see Map 1.1).[1] The early history of the Opelousas Territory is concerned with several Parishes, including Acadia, Evangeline, and
St. Landry, that are the focus of my research. Prior to 1840, these parishes
were all combined as one and known as Imperial St. Landry Parish. Later
Imperial St. Landry was divided and became Calcasieu and St. Landry. Today,
Imperial St. Landry (also known as the original Opelousas Territory) consists
of eight parishes (see Map 1.2). These parishes are: (1) St. Landry, which has
always been considered the mother parish of this region and the seat of the
Opelousas territory; (2) Allen parish, the home of the Koasati American Indians, established in 1912; (3) Evangeline, once the home of a Choctaw settlement established in 1910 (Gahn 1941); (4) Calcasieu, founded in 1840; (5)
Cameron, founded in 1870; (6) Acadia, founded in 1886; and (7) Beauregard,
and (8) Jefferson Davis, both founded in 1912.

These data reveal the demographics of the parishes, then and now, including an overview of the cultural groups of the area, religious institutions in the
area, health conditions, economic conditions, and historical and cultural aspects of the community. Since this study is not a detailed account of the
history of Louisiana's cultural groups, only a preliminary overview is offered.
It is hoped that this preliminary overview will offer some insight into the
effects contact, cross-cultural racial and social mixing, and cultural adaptations
had on the enslaved African.

Map 1.1
Louisiana Parish Map, 1812

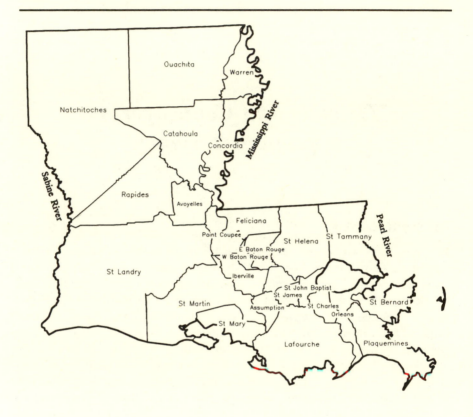

Ouachita

Warren

Natchitoches

Mississippi River

Catahoula

Concordia

Sabine River

Rapides

Avoyelles

Feliciana

Point Coupee

St Helena

St Tammany

Pearl River

E Baton Rouge

W Baton Rouge

St Landry

Iberville

St John Baptist

St James

St Martin

Assumption

St Charles

St Bernard

Orleans

St Mary

Lafourche

Plaquemines

Miles

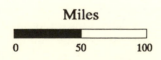

0   50   100

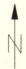

N

Source: Produced by Phil Sheafer.

2

Map 1.3
Native American Linguistic Regions, 1700

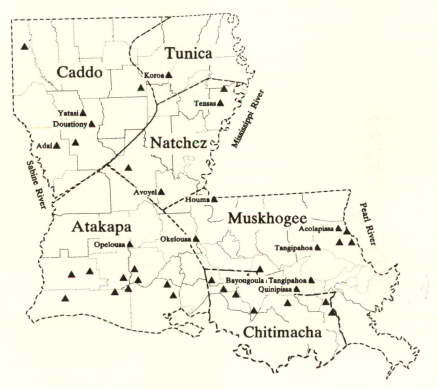

Tunica

Caddo   Koroa ▲

              Tensas ▲

Yatasi ▲
Doustiony ▲

Adai ▲

              Natchez

        Avoyel ▲
              Houma ▲

Atakapa   Muskhogee
                                  Acolapissa ▲
        Opelousa ▲   Okelousa ▲
                            Tangipahoa ▲

              Bayougoula ╷ Tangipahoa ▲
                          Quinipissa ▲

                    Chitimacha

Mississippi River

Sabine River

Pearl River

▲   Native American Communities

---   Linguistic Regions

Miles

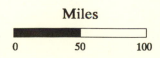

0   50   100

N

Source: Produced by Phil Sheafer.

1919) (See Map 1.4). All of these ethnic groups are language isolates, however. The same diseases, liquor consumption, wars, etc., that affected other North American Native American populations are said to be the maladies which contributed to the demise of the Atakapa and Opelousa.

In general, historic Native Americans in Louisiana were mound builders. Unexplored and explored mounds survive as remnants of Louisiana's historic Native American ethnic groups. Mounds can be found on private property as well as at archeological sites.[4] These mounds were used by the aboriginal to conduct religious ceremonies. Sacred temples were sometimes built on them, and in some cases they served as burial grounds (Kniffen 1987, 259).

The powerful aboriginal Natchez were found in north central Louisiana. They became extinct around 1733 after the French and Natchez war. Those that survived the war and were able to escape French capture merged with the Creek in upper Louisiana and Mississippi. Others that were less fortunate were sold into slavery in Haiti.

In the late 1600s other Native American groups began to migrate to southwest Louisiana. Those who migrated to Louisiana were the Choctaw, Chitimacha, Alabama, and the Koasati. Although the cultural history of the Louisiana aboriginal Indians is scarce, that of the migratory groups is well documented.[5]

The Opelousa were a very friendly, non-warlike people, and it is said that they welcomed the French, who originally came to the region to establish trade. Opelousa means "black head" or "black skull" (Brackenridge 1962). The most *commonly* accepted term is "black foot" or "black leg" (Colliard 1921, 14; Fontenot 1970).

The first record of the Opelousas territory appeared in approximately the late 1690s. The present day city of Opelousas was once inhabited by the Opelousa Native Americans. Full blood Opelousas were last seen in this area around the 1930s. Some African Americans claim Opelousa heritage, and it is also believed that some surviving Opelousa might have mixed with the Bayou Chicot Choctaws. Bayou Chicot is a small town located in Evangeline Parish that was once part of the Opelousas Territory. They also have been identified as Alabamas and are said to be cousins to the Creek (Davis 1806, 97). Their housing was a round tepee-like structure.[6]

The Atakapa, the other aboriginal group of the southwest region, were larger in number than the Opelousa, and they were believed to be man-eaters. This claim to be cannibals and as nomadic is widely debated. Some scholars (Post 1962; Kniffen 1987) believe that cannibalism and nomadic habits were exaggerated. In any case they were friendly with the Opelousas. In 1592, Cabeza de Vaca, one of the early explorers of Louisiana described the Atakapa as tall, well-formed, and brown skinned (Butler 1970). In 1698 there were 3,500 Atakapas in southwest Louisiana, by 1908 there were only nine known survivors (Post 1962). There is an African-American woman in a nearby parish who is part Atakapa.[7]

Map 1.4
Contemporary Native Americans: Language Group Locations and Linguistic Retention

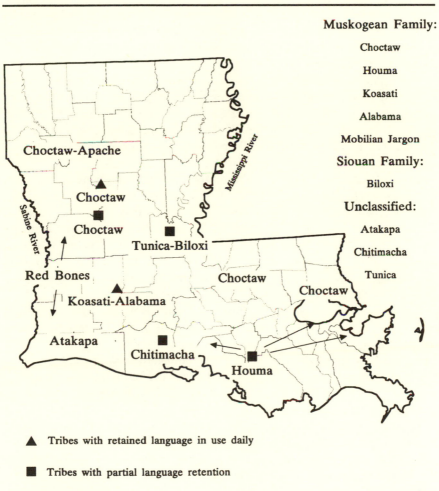

Muskogean Family:

Choctaw

Houma

Koasati

Alabama

Mobilian Jargon

Siouan Family:

Biloxi

Unclassified:

Atakapa

Chitimacha

Tunica

▲ Tribes with retained language in use daily

■ Tribes with partial language retention

Miles

0   50   100

Source: Produced by Phil Sheafer.

The Atakapa villages were found near rivers—the Vermillion and Calcasieu. Their diet consisted of native fruits like persimmons, hickory nuts, and
berries. They mainly survived by fishing, hunting, and raising cattle. Agri-
culture was not a means of subsistence. The Atakapa owned a considerable
amount of cattle, enough so that it was necessary to register their brands
(Post 1962). Because of their habitat and location, the Atakapa were of little
threat to the French. They were not an asset either, and they were not as
friendly with the French as the Opelousa were. The contemporary Native
Americans who settled the southwest region are the Chitimacha, Choctaw,
Alabama, and Koasati.

The Chitimacha, also a language-isolate group, came and settled in the
southwest region along Bayou Teche and the Mississippi River in approximately the early 1700s. They were a people who believed in adorning their
bodies. Men and women wore jewelry, including bracelets, finger rings, and
earrings (Taylor 1979). Their main occupation was originally fishing and they
relied on crops of corn and sweet potatoes.

The early Chitimacha settlement built their homes in a row on bayou banks
and covered them with palmetto leaves. The palmetto plant was also widely
used by other Louisiana Native Americans. It was used in much the same
fashion by African Americans, especially those with Native American heritage,
who say that some of their early homes had roofs made of palmetto plants.
The palmetto root was used for medicinal purposes. The present Chitimacha
are known for their beautiful baskets, and most are employed in the nearby
oil industry outside of Lafayette.

Koasati (Coushattas) belong to the Muskogean language group (Gatschet
1884). The first Koasatis to settle in Louisiana came from Georgia and Alabama
around the late 1700s; in the early 1800s more Coushattas moved from Alabama to Texas and Louisiana. Oral and written records indicate that the Koasatis lived in the present day City of Opelousas in the late 1790s.[8] By the 1850s,
after several moves, the Coushattas settled in Allen Parish just west of St.
Landry; they still are located there.

Today the Koasatis, a warm people, are struggling to maintain their cultural
traditions. While many of the older Koasatis speak only Koasati, the younger
generations are usually bilingual—they speak English and Koasati. Some of
the Koasatis also speak French, because French is a common language for
many older residents of this southwest region. Parts of the Koasati settlement
are surrounded by the local working class African-American community. Other
parts are surrounded by woods and the business district of the town of Elton.
Some of the oral history data that I was able to obtain about the Koasati was
given to me by local African Americans. The Koasatis and the African Americans have been known to intermarry. These mixed blooded African Ameri-
cans/Koasatis can be found in Evangeline, St. Landry, and Allen Parishes.
African Americans and Koasatis also socialize together, conduct business trans-

actions between them, and some members of the African-American community regularly visit the local Koasati church.

According to some Koasati members, they continually struggle to preserve and promote language and cultural pride among the younger generation. This is not an easy task given the influences of television, radio, and peer pressure from the outside, and pressures from insiders who reject tradition and favor western ways. This is one reason why worship services are conducted in Koasati. In addition, the tradition of making pine straw needle baskets is continued, as well as some traditional forms of dance and foods.

The Alabamas originally occupied the northern and western areas in present day St. Landry Parish and parts of present day Evangeline Parish in the late 1700s. Many African-American persons in southwest Louisiana say they have Choctaw and Alabama heritage.

The Choctaws are now found in the northern portions of Louisiana, but in the 1700s they occupied several areas in St. Landry parish around Bayou Chicot.

FRENCH SETTLERS

Louisiana was an infant colony of France. The first and largest group of immigrants who came to the Louisiana colony were men who came directly from France in the early 1700s. French women began to arrive in the colony in significant numbers in the 1720s. The first settlers came as a result of France's efforts to settle the new frontier. They were inspired by land grants offered by the French and Spanish governments. These settlers were upper middle-class Frenchmen who sought opportunities to increase their wealth.

Shortly thereafter, the importation of Africans to be sold as slave laborers began; The Spanish arrived as rulers in the mid 1700s. Later, around 1760, the Cajuns came. French migration from Haiti also had an influence on Louisiana's culture. It started in the late 1700s and continued until the early 1800s. Other European groups also came to Louisiana, but their cultural influence and numbers were not as great.

Early African-American communities in this region played a major role in the development of the area culturally and economically. In Grand Prairie, Leonville, Plaisance, and Palmetto, for example, we have old land gentried African-American families. These are some of the oldest farm settlements and four of the oldest Black farm communities dating back to the 1700s (Myers 1987; Fontenot 1988).

Settlement in the Opelousas Territory began in 1717, when John Law, a Scotsman, was granted a charter that stipulated he bring 1,500 settlers and 3,000 enslaved Africans to the land granted him (Thistlethwaite 1970, 33). The original settlers of the Opelousas territory were cattle grazers who owned from 1,000 to 3,000 heads of cattle. Later, less emphasis was placed on cattle raising, and early settlers began to farm the very fertile land. The early land claimants included whites as well as Free Persons of Color. Both ethnic groups had to meet the ordinance requirements—slave and stock ownership—in order to claim land (Oubre 1973).

Acquiring land grants was also a means utilized by white fathers to emancipate their mulatto sons. These fathers sent their sons to the Opelousas frontier to start cattle farms, and in return for their services the sons received freedom and stock. The French acquired land in other ways also. Some land was purchased from the Atakapa Indians, some was obtained by order of survey issued by the governor, and by occupation, later confirmed by the government (Griffin 1959).

In 1769 about one hundred families lived in Opelousas. By 1776 there were 139 families. The population began to increase due to the Spanish Land Grant Policy, which stated that a person was eligible to claim the forty acre land grant if he or she owned a substantial number of cattle and livestock and owned at least two slaves (enslaved Africans). This policy was only partly responsible for the increased number of residents in the parish. Additionally, the increased population was due to the migration of French military persons to St. Landry from Alabama and France and the arrival of other Anglo-Americans from other American colonies. By the end of the 1700s, Louisiana was pretty well established; then came the sale in 1803.

The Haitian revolution of 1803, in which Toussaint l'Ouverture, an African, led a group of Voodoo worshipers in the overthrow of French rule in Haiti, was one of the key reasons France sold the Louisiana territory to the United States. This sale price of $15,000,000 for about one million square miles of land, averaged four cents a square mile (Chidsey 1972; LaFargue 1940). Louisiana remained the territory of the United States until it became a state in 1812.

When Louisiana changed hands to the English Americans, a great deal of resentment existed among Louisiana French residents toward the new owners (Robertson 1969). The new American government was not welcome. Those unfavorable attitudes existed in the Opelousas territory, as well as in the New Orleans area. Elisha Bowman, an early Methodist minister, had this to say about the people in the Opelousas region, "I find the people very much dissatisfied with the American government and we have a constant talk of war . . . three-fourths of the people hope they will get this country again. . . . Three-fourths of the inhabitants of this country, I suppose, are French" (Fontenot 1970, 29).

The Americanization of Louisiana was a slow process; France had left her mark on Louisiana. Even today Louisiana's culture has a strong French influence; French language and customs prevail, including a judicial system based on the Napoleon Code instead of the English common Law, and a French form of government. The immigration of Black French persons into Louisiana after the Haitian revolution also contributed to the maintenance of French Caribbean and African cultural traditions (Hunt 1988). This migration continued until the early 1800s and is one reason Louisiana has been referred to as a Caribbean Island.

The Americans were aware of the resistant attitudes of Louisiana's residents of French ancestry. In an effort to make the transition from a French to an American government a harmonious one, they allowed certain aspects of the cultural traditions to remain, such as the legal system. By 1804 however, English was introduced as the official language in legislative matters (Newton 1929). The use of English as an official language became an issue in rural southwest Louisiana again in the late 1950s. Today, there is a continuous concerted effort on the part of many contemporary cultural revivalists to reintroduce French in the schools and community.

SPANISH RULE

The period of Spanish rule in Louisiana, 1763 to 1803, is one aspect of Louisiana history that is often ignored. There are however many contributions made by the Spanish to the history of Louisiana. For example, traces of Spanish heritage can be found in architecture, foods, and surnames like Donatto, Martinez, Perez, etc. Cuba was the Spanish administrative seat governing Louisiana, so most of the early Spanish people who settled in Louisiana came from there (Morazan 1983).

CAJUN ARRIVAL

Another group, known as Cajuns—descendants from Canada who were the victims of expulsion—settled in the eastern and southern portion of the southwest area (Dormon 1983). Most came to Louisiana, via Haiti, around 1760. Unlike the early French settlers of the area, Cajuns' early life in the southwest region was one of poverty and isolation. Very few owned slaves, and interaction with Africans was limited. They were granted subsistence and permitted to settle in the old Atakapa region by Denis-Nicolas Foucault, then Commissaire-Oronnateur of Louisiana, because the Cajuns were impoverished and needed charity (Brasseaux 1975). The original Cajun settlers and their descendants mainly occupy the present parishes of St. Mary, St. Martin, Lafayette, Iberia, and Vermillion.

THE AFRICAN EXPERIENCE

Important dates for African Americans in this area are 1712, 1720, and 1724. The first ship of Africans arrived in Louisiana around 1712. By 1720, French land grantees began to settle the Opelousas frontier, bringing with them enslaved Africans. Some of the settlers included Louisiana's first mixed bloods—mulattoes.[9]

The early severe climatic conditions—humidity, heat, and mosquitos—still existant today, proved to be devastating to the early French and Spanish set-tlers. So, African slaves were brought to the area, and their labor was used to build the colony and work the sugarcane, cotton, and indigo fields. Early slave owners were both Black and White; most having fewer than twenty slaves, however.

The slaves came from many West African countries, as was the case in most of the Americas. Gwendolyn Midlo Hall and other scholars confirm that the first Africans to arrive in Louisiana came from Senegal, Gambia, and the Congo.[10] Many were Bambaras from the empire of Mali, West Africa (Taylor 1963). The summer of 1719 marked the arrival of five hundred Africans from Guinea. In the year 1721, slave ships brought Africans from Senegal, and some Africans are reported to have come from the Congo (Dart 1931b). However, by 1726, most Africans that were brought to Louisiana were Bambaras and Senegalese.

The Senegalese were favored by the French for their skill and expertise as farmers, and the French were especially interested in the Senegalese talents with growing rice. As a growing colony, Louisiana needed to establish an economic base. The French colonizers had hoped that the farming expertise of the Senegalese, combined with the commercialization of rice, indigo, and tobacco, would provide them with the labor and profits needed to establish an economic foundation. The French were also partial to the Senegalese be-cause they did not rebel as frequently as the Bambara (also noted for their farming expertise), nor were the Senegalese as inclined to run away from the plantation as were the Gambians.

In some ways the exploitation of slave labor resulted in the artistic expres-sion of the enslaved African and the creation of a class of major Black artisans in Louisiana. In New Orleans, evidence of black craftsmanship is visible in the French Quarter with its beautiful iron works found on balconies, gates, etc. (Christian 1972).

Another relic of early West African culture and craftsmanship is the African House built in 1750. This house is located in the southwest region and was built under the supervision of a Free Woman of Color, Marie Metoyer, who came from Ghana. It is called an African House because of its architectural design, which is similar to the design concept of West African houses.

Indeed, the first enslaved Africans became the early blacksmiths, carpen-ters, locksmiths, sculptors, masons, and bricklayers in Louisiana. Much of these same skills are highly respected occupations among the African-Amer-ican working-class population today. In rural communities, such as the Ope-lousas region, African Americans boast about their ability or the ability of relatives to build family residences. Some of these family homes date back to the 1800s.

These early skills created a class all its own, separate and apart from the freed or the enslaved populations, although many persons in the free popu-lation possessed talent as carpenters, etc. These kinds of occupations created close working conditions between Blacks and Whites and often resulted in emancipation (Usner 1979).

The most important set of laws implemented during the colonial period, which would have a lasting influence on the traditions of Africans, were Le Codes Noir (The Black Codes). These laws were initially formulated for the French West Indies in 1685, and in 1724 modified for Louisiana (Allain 1980). They were severe regulations, or police policies (fifty-five of them), especially written for people of African descent and were responsible for the beginning of a police control of sorts, often cruel and barbarous. They restricted movement, controlled economic growth, and placed lowered economic value on property owned by persons of African descent.

The Codes have been described as paternalistic rather than designed to enforce slavery and racial prejudice (rules and guidelines for parents to follow when governing and disciplining their children). The Codes are said to reflect the French monarchy's attitude toward order, unity, and the desire to make Louisiana more like the motherland, France (Allain 1980).

In reality these Codes were primarily concerned with (1) the enslaved African as property, and ways and means by which to protect that investment; (2) providing the complete and watchful control of Free People of Color; and (3) enforcing Catholicism as the main religion (which played a part in influencing present day syncretic folk medicine and religious traditions of Louisiana African Americans).

The most significant Articles, one and two, of the Codes introduced Catholicism into the West Indies and Louisiana in the mid 1720s. These Codes reflected absolute control and demanded religious unity believed to be necessary for civil peace. The first order of business was to convert enslaved Africans to Catholicism. African slaves were baptized in Christian ceremonies. Those that were baptized were in most cases eventually buried in Christian cemeteries.

In the early 1700s the Black population begin to outnumber Whites. This was partly due to the increase of mixed-blood children of African, French, and Indian ancestry. Fear that freed Blacks and mulatto children would gain the sympathy of French allies developed. In an effort to curtail the growing population of free Blacks, one article of the Code stipulated that cohabitation between French men and women of African descent would no longer be tolerated and thus became illegal. The famous Code Noir, often ignored by Whites, dealt:

mainly with slaves, though it also restricted the privileges of free Negroes. It required Catholic instruction and baptism for all slaves; forbade marriage or concubinage of white or free born or manumitted Negroes with slaves; fixed the conditions by which slaves could marry; deprived slaves of the right to sue or be sued; forbade the shackling of slaves; declared Negroes movable property; stated the conditions under which they might be manumitted and regulated in great detail the manner in which slaves might be punished. (Griffin 1959, 30)

During the early years of the Code Noir, many French slaveholders were relaxed about following these regulations. Interracial marriages and cohabitation continued, manumission occurred, and public gatherings among enslaved and freed Africans were permitted between plantations and at the homes of free Blacks.

The lack of a sufficient number of White women in the colony made it difficult to restrict cohabitation between French men and African women. Insufficient numbers of available mates were also partly the reason for continued marriages between free persons and enslaved persons of color. Often marriages between freed and enslaved populations were for the purposes of liberty. Free Persons of Color were thus in a position to work out agreements with slave owners in which they would purchase the freedom of their spouse or relative, further increasing the number of freed persons.

The French are said to have been the most lenient of the slaveholders throughout the colonies of the Americas; this was due to Article 43 of the Code Noir, which specified that enslaved families with children under the age of fourteen should be kept together and not sold separately. Surprisingly this was faithfully enforced in many of the cases involving slave sales. Africans were encouraged to utilize their time off on Sundays to sell goods, or hire out, to bring in extra income for themselves and their families. One can see how it was possible for blacks in Louisiana, unlike other areas in the South, to purchase their freedom and the freedom of their loved ones.

By the year 1751 policies to control the slave population were strictly enforced, and Louisiana begin to move more toward a state where slaves were viewed as incorrigible. Runaways were on the increase. They fled to wooded areas and bayou country where they organized with other runaways and remained uncaptured. They survived by joining Native American settlements and by looting plantations on the Mississippi. Slaveholders became alarmingly concerned about the growing population of slaves who remained at large. The Codes in essence, changed the lifestyle of Blacks in Louisiana (Brasseaux 1980); they remained in effect until 1806 when they were revised by the Territory of Orleans.

A totalitarian form of government ruled until 1845 when a Jacksonian democratic process begin in this area. Prior to 1845, voting privileges were extended to only landed gentry White males twenty-one and over who owned fifty acres of land or more. In 1845 a new constitution went into effect and the common man (white men), twenty-one and over, was enfranchised to vote. Local officials were now elected by popular vote, whereas before officials were appointed by the Governor or state legislation. Blacks and women however were still ineligible to vote. Immediately after the Civil War persons of African descent were allowed to vote, and some were elected state legislators, until 1989. Nonetheless, in 1898 a Louisiana constitutional law known as the "Grandfather Clause" was instituted that would alter voting privileges of

Blacks. Article 197 (Grandfather Clause) of the constitution mandated that Black residents could not vote because their grandfathers did not vote.

When it comes to the vote, Blacks have always been a political pawn in this rural area. One White interviewee stated that a local Free Man of Color was convinced to sell his political position to a White in the late 1800s causing disruption in the Black community.[11] Between 1830 and 1860 Free People of Color (FPC) were allowed to vote in certain elections, if it meant the FPC's vote would help a White candidate win an election. This issue of buying votes from Blacks who were recognized leaders in the Black community created much deception and division among Blacks.

There were continued attempts and scare tactics by St. Landry Parish Whites to force Blacks into acquiescence. White hate groups tried to introduce a state ordinance that would reduce the Free People of Color population to a status of semi-slavery. If the Colored free person was convicted of a crime, for example, instead of having the same sentencing as any other White free person, he or she was to be sold back into slavery for life. The selling of liquor to the enslaved African population by a Free Person of Color was also to be forbidden—it was to be considered an act to incite rioting and the punishment was also to be re-enslavement. Fortunately, these legislative attempts never succeeded (Sterkx 1972).

The general attitude toward the emancipation of the Negro in 1865 was a bitter one. The race riot in St. Landry parish of that same year illustrates this. One account states that although the Whites of St. Landry condoned the defeat of slavery, they didn't want ex-slaves to rule them (Dupre 1970). The general attitude of vigilante Whites then became one of malice, and a deliberate plan was devised to oppress Blacks to assure subserviency. Their plan included the hanging of many early Black political leaders involved with issues centered around emancipation (DeLatte 1976).

CONTEMPORARY COMMUNITY

The Opelousas Territory is located in the western and south-central part of Louisiana and mainly consists of a vast prairie. The prairie area has a very humid, subtropical climate with an average rainfall of fifty-seven inches annually. Winter and spring are the best times to visit for those unaccustomed to the hot, humid summer and fall months. July and August are the hottest months, with frequent heatwaves.

Hurricanes and tornadoes are common happenings in Louisiana, and they often leave destructive paths. Bayous, rivers, swamps, and marshes dominate the eastern and southern portion of the southwest area. Familiar flora and fauna in the area consist of palmettoes in the swamp areas; pecan groves, live oak, and the very useful and durable cypress trees around the marsh areas.[12] Fruits such as fig, peach, watermelon, and plums are plentiful. Many locals still savor the locally wild grown muskedine grape.[13] Historically, fishing as a

Secret Doctors

means of subsistence has always been popular, and this is still the case today. Louisiana is known as "sportsmen paradise," and the state automobile license plate advertises this slogan. Many trappers, hunters, and fishermen seek out game, such as the native alligators and the popular crayfish, as food staples. Woody areas are in abundance and wild game remains a means of food supply for many, including African Americans, who regularly hunt rabbit, squirrel, deer, and various birds. Local farmers often complain about the foxes and coyotes that frequently make their supper of the farmers "yard chickens."

The Opelousas region was once a major center for commercial and governmental activity in Louisiana, with the cities of Opelousas, Washington, and Port Barre, being the seat of the activities. This region, and the New Orleans area, in particular are prideful of their French heritage. One can find many African and French cultural traits throughout the area. The food of African Americans is one way in which the broader culture has been influenced. Although the herb "file" is of Native American origin, the use of okra in a file gumbo is believed to be of African origin. The word gumbo (a souplike dish) is also said to be of African origin.

The Opelousas region is bilingual. The population speaks English as well as several creolized dialects of French. The African Americans have their pidgin, the Euro-French have theirs, and the Cajuns have their own. All are descendants of some of the first settlers, and each acquired a vernacular of French as their first language, based on their individual cultural heritage (Butler 1969; Hymes 1971; Tentchoff 1975; Rickford 1977; Smitherman 1977; Valdman 1977, 1983). Social and cultural activities, as well as family stories, also reflect African, Native American, French, Spanish, and Cajun heritages.

This region is unique in that it is an area fast becoming the second leading tourist attraction in Louisiana. This is primarily because of Louisiana's cultural heritage and the extensive promotional efforts being carried out to promote the southwest area. Afro-Creole and Cajun food, Zydeco (African-derived) and Cajun music (European-derived), mysterious landscapes of swamps, bayous, and the subtropical climate all contribute to the uniqueness of the area. These were characteristics taken for granted just a few years ago.

The southwestern Louisiana people are proud of their social and business connections with Canada and France, and these countries maintain business and cultural commitments to the area as well. Additionally, there are cultural, business, and educational alliance programs between residents of Louisiana, Canada, and France. The alliance between Afro-French and Afro-Haitian heritages is recognized in part through a symposium by the University of Southwestern Louisiana sponsoring visiting French West Indian artists and scholars. Local clubs and organizations were also organized for the promotion and preservation of French African-American traditions. Other efforts are being made to maintain the French connection. The local and state governments, for example, are carrying out cultural and legislative activities designed to promote the French heritage of the area. The French language, after seventy years, is being revived and reinstated in schools (in 1921 state legislation mandated that only English was to be spoken in schools).

The approximate total population for all three parishes is 183,000, with a total farm population of approximately 99,000. African Americans make up about 60,000 of the tri-parish area. There is a small percentage of Vietnamese, but documents are inaccessible. Most of the old African-American secret doctors/treaters are from isolated rural farm municipalities with populations of 600 or less. Others are from rural townships where the population is 3,000 or less, and some are from rural urban towns where the population is under 19,000.

ECONOMIC CONDITIONS

In the early 1700s the economy in the St. Landry region was based on cattle raising and agricultural hinterlands. The major crops were tobacco, indigo, and corn; secondary crops were rice and sugarcane. Cotton and yams came into demand in the late 1800s. The present economy also has an agricultural base—primarily sweet potatoes and soybeans.

Presently, the economy is depressed, due mainly to the collapse of the oil industry located in the city of Lafayette, the oil center of Louisiana. Louisiana was a major site for the U.S. oil industries and relied heavily on the oil trade prior to the decline of oil production in the early 1980s. Many people have relocated to other areas as a result of the industry's decline.

This region has the second largest rural population in the state. The median family income is $13,893. Louisiana has one of the highest unemployment rates in the United States, and St. Landry Parish has the highest unemployed population in the state; even the farming economy is not stable. In 1980 the gross income for agriculture in the Parish was $89 million; by 1987 that amount fell to $56 million. Farming, nonetheless, remains the major source of income for the parish (Normand 1989).

At present the parish population is diminishing on an average of 2% yearly. This is due to the poor economy and lack of employment opportunities, especially for African Americans. Twenty percent of the African Americans, compared to seven percent of the White population, are leaving the area in search of better, and equal, employment opportunities. Once college-educated, opportunities for professional African Americans are limited locally, except as teachers, principals, or other employment related to secondary education; even these jobs are few in number.

Professional and paraprofessional positions are simply not open to the masses of African Americans in this community. Black men are the highest percent of the unemployed and underemployed population. Many African Americans, both literate and illiterate, are paid minimum wage or they are underpaid. The largest African-American workforce remains in farming, or farm-related labor. Some African Americans own their own farms, some are tenant farmers, and a large percentage are hired out as domestic, field, and common laborers.

In a State Department of Labor survey for the Parishes of St. Landry, Evangeline, and Acadia, Whites hold 421 of the professional medical and health care positions (i.e., doctors, nurses, social workers, etc.) while Blacks hold 105. Teaching by far is the area with the highest percentage of Black professionals. Out of 1,814 teaching jobs, 813 are held by blacks and 1,001 are held by Whites; 625 of those teaching positions are Black women and 734 are White women. In domestic and cleaning services Black women and men are most often found in these jobs; 390 Black women perform private household duties in contrast to seventy-seven White women (Bartels 1989).

POLITICAL SYSTEM

During the colonial period, the political structure of the Opelousas region, and other parts of the Louisiana territory, was a military (Commandants) form of government. Orders were received from at various times the Governor General of Paris, the Viceroy of Cuba, and the King of Spain. Civil official appointments by the Governor began in 1805. Between 1807 and 1819 the parishes were formed. Thus began the "Anglo-American" jurisprudence form of government, placed on top of a French political system and attitude already in existence.

The involvement of African Americans in the political process in Louisiana gradually decreased during the middle and late 1800s. African Americans, including some Native Americans, were allowed to vote from the end of the Civil War until 1896. They did not vote again until the early 1950s (Fontenot 1970).

Prior to the 1960s voting eligibility for Blacks in Louisiana was determined based upon how much Blacks knew about the structure of government on the local, state, and national levels. "To prove they knew about current political events Blacks were required to pass a written test based on historical and contemporary, political and governmental issues."[14] Neither Black nor White women were eligible to vote; however, they could own property and could lawfully maintain that property separate and apart from their husbands, if married.

The forms of government and/or leadership roles that exist in the cities of this tri-parish area today are similar to that of other cities. African Americans and women have made contributions in leadership roles. The mayor in Opelousas is an African American, and he serves as the first elected Black Mayor for the city; however, other Blacks in the region also hold this office. The Clerk of Court is another elected position in the city. The person in this position is responsible for maintaining court records and legal documents. Recently a woman was elected as clerk, another first for the area.

Each city in the parish has a City Council. Blacks hold some of these elected positions. The number of council members for each city depends on the parish district's land area and number of inhabitants. This governing body is responsible for providing the city residents with all public services, for example, electricity, water, etc.

One of the surviving French forms of governing bodies is the Police Juror, first organized about 1811. Some members of this governing body are African Americans. Initially this was an elected-at-large position. Following several disputes about the election process, and a recent legal battle between White and African-American community members, elections for these positions are now based on vote by distribution. This is a very politically powerful governing body whose main responsibility is the construction, repair, and maintenance of drainage systems and parish roads. In an area where flooding is a constant concern, one can understand why a Police Juror is an important "political" figure in the community.

The parishes' school boards consist of elected members representing the various political districts in each Parish. St. Landry has a Black school board president, another first for the parish.

RELIGION

The two dominant religious denominations are Catholic and Baptist. Most of the African Americans in the region are Baptist. However, the influence of Catholicism in Louisiana is central to the religious thinking of the people. Prior to the early 1800s, Catholicism in the Opelousas region, like most of Louisiana, was the only legalized religion. Persons were not required to attend worship services, but "public respect and acknowledgement of Catholicism as the only faith was expected" (Davis 1806, 55).

The first church in the area was the White St. Landry Catholic Church established in 1774 in Washington, Louisiana; the church later moved to Opelousas. It was not until the 1830s that churches of other denominations began to take root. The exception to this were the Baptist churches started by African Americans. Records show that Calvary Baptist and Canaan Baptist, both Black churches, were organized in the early 1800s; however, most Black Baptist churches blossomed in the mid 1860s and thereafter. The first White Baptist church was organized in late 1880. The first Black Catholic church in the Opelousas region was organized in 1920. Black Catholic churches in the other area were organized between the 1940s and 1950s.

In 1812 Calvary Baptist church in Bayou Chicot was the first Black Baptist church in Louisiana, and the first west of the Mississippi. It was established in the Opelousas territory, in what is now known as Evangeline parish, by a Free Person of Color, Joseph Willis. Beginning early in the 1800s, religious rebellion and community organizing via the African-American church began under the direction of leaders from Free Persons of Color communities like Joseph Willis (Fitts 1985).

Willis, from South Carolina, went to Louisiana for the purpose of minister-
ing to the Opelousa Native Americans in 1804. He then began to minister to
persons of African descent. The success Willis achieved in establishing an
African-American Church at that time will perhaps never fully be understood.
Many oral accounts relate stories of vigilante groups who destroyed church
structures and made it difficult for Black persons who were attempting to start
their own churches.[15] In any case this was a time of political turmoil in Louisiana. She was seeking statehood, and there was debate as to whether Louisiana should be admitted to the Union. Perhaps the confusion of statehood
and the general feelings that Willis' religious organizing efforts were not detrimental to the masses of the state helped paved the path for his success.
Furthermore, church organizing was a pattern established in other states
among Blacks in Protestant denominations.

According to oral history accounts, African Americans were "having church
in each other's homes, praying and praising God" long before the 1860s.[16] One
female elder of the local African-American community said, "We were having
church long before that. Our parents used to tell us how they had to hide and
meet in houses to hold prayer meetings."[17] What began as prayer meetings
were in actuality formalized church worship. Perhaps this is the case for many
early Black churches, although there are no formal records. Perhaps what
started as efforts to conceal their church existence, has resulted in missing
data and gaps in history about early African-American Christian worship styles
and traditions. Early formal records were not maintained, and Blacks were
very secretive about announcing worship meetings. As a result, many of the
churches have a history older than what is documented.

Blacks attended local White Catholic churches until the early 1900s when
Black Catholic churches began to flourish. When Blacks attended services at
these churches they sat in the rear and in the "galleys" (balconies). Some
even rented benches (designated by the church for those Blacks who could
afford them) that were placed in the rear and reserved for a particular Black
person or family. There is an old saying in the community that "all Blacks
in Louisiana were born Catholic" (meaning they were all Catholics before
they became any other Christian denomination). Many African Americans today maintain the graves of their early ancestors who are buried in White
Catholic church cemeteries.[18] Even though Blacks could not participate in
Catholic church worship services, or activities, they were encouraged by
Whites to attend local White churches.

The mandatory attendance of Blacks in White Catholic churches continued
until the 1940s. Growing discontent mounted against Blacks who continued
to frequent White churches. White church attenders complained that Blacks,
who were very vocal with shouts and other charismatic forms of worship, were
too noisy as worshipers. Gradually Blacks were discouraged from attending,

and adequate facilities for Black Catholics were fully provided in the mid 1900s (May 1981).

LITERACY

Illiteracy remains a problem in this community among all ethnic groups, but it is extremely high among this rural African-American population. It is equal in proportion among the old and the young.

The first White public school opened in 1871 in Washington, Louisiana. During the formative years of education in the region, emphasis was placed on educating young White women. Some students received tutoring, and some were sent to the Opelousas Female Academy which opened its doors in 1850. Early Black families likewise stressed education for their young daughters.

Public education for Blacks in Louisiana had its beginnings in the mid 1800s, in what was known as "Church Schools" (Eakin 1980). These were schools founded, operated, and funded by local Black Baptist churches. Many of these church schools (Truevine, Mohorn, and New Bethel, for example) held classes in small buildings constructed on the church grounds for that purpose, or classes were held in the church temple. The land needed to build these Black churches and church schools was in most cases donated by a Black church member.

In 1920 a separate church parish was established for Black Catholics; shortly thereafter Holy Ghost Catholic School was founded and became the first Black Catholic school to be accredited by the State.

After 1910 state-supported public school education for African Americans in rural areas began. Although early state public schools were considered property of the parish, the African-American community often raised their own funds to build new buildings or acquire supplies for teaching and learning (Jones 1980). Very few resources were provided during these early times by what was then a white ruling school board.

All of these predominately Black schools (including Holy Ghost Catholic school) no longer exist. The Supreme Court decisions that were a result of the activities of the Civil Rights movement are responsible for an integration plan that stripped Black public schools of African-American names; Black high schools were reclassified as elementary or junior high schools; and in many cases, Black principals were demoted to status as assistant principals or as principals of elementary schools.

The education issue has been and remains an emotionally bitter issue among African Americans in the area. It also appears that this is the area where African Americans are politically weak. The African-American community complains that African-American educational issues are not a priority, nor a concern, of the mainstream governing body. Hence the educational system, its hiring practices, and overall treatment of African Americans remains a source of major dissatisfaction.[19]

COLOR AND CLASS AMONG AFRICAN AMERICANS

Like urban New Orleans, this rural southwest region has a complex class structure among African Americans. In this instance class is determined by land ownership, occupation, and color. What is significant about this class structure, in relation to this study, is that folk doctors cross all class lines; therefore, class distinctions, as well as family kindreds, among folk doctors often play an important role in determining the social class of his or her patients.

The upper and middle classes are usually persons who descend from a line of landowners and/or have FPC ancestry. Descendants of Free People of Color are divided into two classes—the upper and middle. This is followed by the occupational or working class, and then there is the lower class.

The height of importance of this Free People of Color class formation was between 1724 and about 1780. Although small in number, they were the founders and builders, for the most part, of this African-American culture base. They are responsible for establishing an economic base, a social stratification system, a class structure, and intra-group prejudices based on skin color. These factors left a lasting effect on race and class issues in Louisiana.

There are several Negroid racial mixtures in Louisiana that are relative to this region.

The offspring of a White parent and a Negro parent is a Mulatto (one half white and one half black). The offspring of a White parent and a Mulatto parent is a quarterone or quadroon (three quarters White and one quarter Black). The offspring of a White parent and a quarterone parent is an octoroon (seven eights White and one eight Black). The offspring of a Mulatto parent and a Negro parent is a griffe (one quarter White and three quarters Black). (Leonard and Oubre 1983, 75)

The most frequently used terms to describe someone with African ancestry in Colonial Opelousas territory were Negro, Mulatto, and Quarterone. From 1803 until the 1860s the terms Negro, Mulatto, and Free Person of Color became the terms found in most legal records. A Free Person of Color was any freed person with African blood, regardless of skin color or racial mixture.

There are two communities found among descendants of the Free People of Color social-class population. Persons from both communities are descendants of some of the first settlers (African, French/Spanish, and/or Native American). This FPC class laid the foundation for early African-American upper-class status in Louisiana. One community is composed of primarily light-skinned persons. Many times they go to extremes to assure that the skin color of family descendants remains light from generation to generation. Marriage to another person of a similar color hue appears to be more important for this group than economics (Jones 1950). For the most part this practice remains today.

Another community of persons of the Free People of Color social class population includes persons whose skin hue varies from very light to very dark skinned. Marrying someone of the same hue is not as important as marrying someone on the same economic level. Land ownership for this group (and for the first group) is important. Most land is inherited and has been a part of the family estate in some cases since the 1700s.

The middle class (including persons from mixed heritage) are persons whose lineage is from a group who worked and saved to purchase land. In some cases they were migrants from other states in the original American colonies. As one woman identified a fellow neighbor, "he is a pure American," meaning he does not have French ancestry or is not from French territory.[20] Usually their land acquisition occurred after 1865.

Another class of African Americans (including, in some cases, those from mixed heritage) are those whose parentage are from the occupational or working class. In the rural areas these were people who were house servants or drivers (chauffeurs). Some were brick layers, carpenters, etc. They usually don't own acres of land; instead they may own a home and lot. Their descendants still carry similar type of occupational status.

Some of the same occupations that were popular among early rural Africans are considered the more meaningful skilled trades for persons today. In 1850 the occupational class in rural Louisiana consisted of eighteen Black and 148 Mulatto carpenters, three Black and forty-four Mulatto masons, two Black and eleven Mulatto merchants, two Black and five Mulatto shoemakers, and seven Mulatto butchers. Among the middle and upper classes were one Black and two Mulatto teachers, and one each of Black and Mulatto doctors (Sterkx 1972, 224). Most college-educated persons are from the second sub-class of Free People of Color and from the middle class. The lower class in this region are persons whose roots stem from the field laborers during the plantation era, or whose ancestors were the tenant or sharecropper class. Their descendants, in most cases, still live as renters or tenant farmers.

HOMESTEAD AND LAND OWNERSHIP

Homesteaders in this community are the backbone of the class structure. After emancipation the value of the property of many Black landowners decreased. Names such as "Coon Town" were given to describe predominately Black sections of town in tax rolls and receipts so as to discourage the purchase of the property by Whites (Falanga 1989).

The same tactics used to rob Blacks of their land in the late 1800s and early 1900s are being used by the establishment today to acquire Black land and to discourage Black homesteads. Some of the tactics responsible for Black homesteaders losing their property were back taxes, foreclosure, discriminatory marketing practices, and unfair market value sales.[21]

Despite the difficulties encountered by early Black homesteaders, much of Black land ownership flourished post-emancipation. Thus land gentried Blacks were born pre-emancipation. The desire to homestead was one thing, but the means by which to do so was another. Many post-emancipation freed Blacks had little or no tools, nor the provisions to maintain themselves and their families while they attempted to homestead. Hence in many cases, becoming a landowner was difficult if not impossible (Oubre 1970).

The struggle to maintain land, once acquired, remains a concern for Black homesteaders; as economic conditions worsen and large farmers monopolize the market, more and more Black homesteaders are pushed into bankruptcy and extinction. In 1920, there were 926,000 Black farmers who owned about 15 million acres of farm land. In 1969 there were only 87,000 Black farmers, with less than 6 million acres (Martin 1985).

NOTES

1. For historical information pertaining to the Opelousas Territory, I relied on data from Parish archives and library research. Housed in the St. Landry Parish Court House are old worn records, often hand scripted and in old French. Many of the historical and contemporary data in this study focus on St. Landry Parish since numerous older settlements were in this Parish and most of the historical records of Acadia and Evangeline Parishes can be found in the St. Landry Parish repository. At the Parish archives I examined Parish lawsuits, early maps, conveyance, church, marriage, emancipation, succession, probate records, and plat books, for general information relating to the historical events of the area and the historical events which affected the lives of African Americans in the area.

Several interviews with Clerk of Court officials were conducted to obtain information about early settlers of the Opelousas Territory. In addition, I interviewed elderly Black and White members of the community who offered some local oral history accounts related to social conditions and the relationship between African-Americans and Anglo-Americans in this region during the 1800s and early 1900s. Other interviews were conducted, in person and by telephone, with public health officials, Parish and Federal agricultural agents, secondary and post-secondary academicians, and other nonspecific community members.

I compiled historical data from libraries at Louisiana State University (Baton Rouge); Tulane University (New Orleans); Louisiana State Library (Baton Rouge); University of Southwestern Louisiana (Lafayette); local community Public Libraries; Louisiana Land Grant Office (Baton Rouge); and Chamber of Commerce Offices and Parish Tourism Offices.

2. The original Atakapa region included the present day parishes of Lafayette, St. Martin, Vermillion, Iberia, and St. Mary.

3. Washington was once called Negroville because of the large number of African Americans who settled there.

4. A couple of community private property owners claim that some of these mounds exist on their property.

5. The following sources offer detailed accounts of these Native Americans. They are Bossu 1771; Bushnell 1909; Hudson 1975; Peterson 1975; and Swanton 1911, 1922, 1946.

6. A photo in the Souvenir Edition of the *Daily World*, June 12, 1970, shows this type of housing, believed to exist around 1720.

7. Interview with John Fox, October 1990, Lake Charles, Louisiana.

8. Folklore collection #109, University of Southwestern Louisiana, Folklore Archives Lafayette.

9. Important sources for early history of African Americans in Louisiana in general, and in the southwest region specifically, are Desdunes 1937, DeVille 1973, Kendall 1941, Marc de Villiers 1982, Rousseve 1937, and Sanders 1931.

10. A recent historical study of the African presence in Louisiana was done by Gwendolyn Midlo Hall, *Africans in Colonial Louisiana* (Baton Rouge: Louisiana State University Press, 1992). Congolese heritage is prevalent throughout the Americas (e.g., New Orleans, Haiti, and Brazil). Another area where Congo folk traditions survive is Panama. See Patricia Lund Drolet, "The Congo Ritual of Northeastern Panama: An Afro-American Expressive Structure of Cultural Adaptation" (Ph.D. diss., University of Illinois at Urbana-Champaign, 1980).

11. Interview with Mr. Francois Nuex, October 1988, Opelousas, Louisiana.

12. Because of its durability and adaptation to the humid weather, cypress wood is still cherished as a good wood for building homes.

13. Locals eat these grapes fresh, make preserve with them, or they make traditional muskedine wine.

14. Interview with Black community leader Mr. J. J. Ertip, July 25, 1989, Washington, Louisiana.

15. Interviews with Brothers John Talazo and Frederick Flowers, deacons of a local Baptist church, August 23, 1989, in Ville Plate and Opelousas Louisiana.

16. Interview with Sister Victoria Sauls, deaconess of a local Baptist church, August 9, 1989, Washington, Louisiana.

17. Interview with Sister Olster Domingue, October 13, 1989, Lebeau, Louisiana.

18. Interviews with local community members, Mr. Fudge Jos and Mrs. Mame Sammuels, Washington and Opelousas, Louisiana, October 13, 1988 and September 19, 1988, respectively.

19. Interview with Mr. Howard Morganza, November 1988, Opelousas Louisiana.

20. Interview conducted with Mrs. L. Tissey, February 29, 1990, Eunice, Louisiana.

21. Many oral history accounts cite instances where Black land owners lost their land because of illegal tax debts.

2

African Americans and Medicine: A Historical Perspective

"Yes I still go see 'Treaters'[1] for some things," Bae Bae said. "Like my boy had been complaining about pain in his stomach and his privates, so I took him to see a Treater for . . . that ailment. What you call that Shae? That's kinda like when children go through, or like when we [women] go through our cycle," she continued.

"Oh, like puberty?" I asked.

"Yea!" Shae responded enthusiastically. "But the boys go through something different. The growing they call that. Its just like the growing, but you have to say that in French, that's the right way. You call that the 'grandeur' that means growing." "So I took him to see the treater," Bae Bae said, "because no [sic] White doctor understand that. And besides I was scared to take him to see one. That's such a private thing. I didn't want him messed up for life" [implying she didn't trust a White doctor examining her son's sexual organs]. Continuing she said, "Then he (secret doctor) give me a gallon of some medicine called 'teezon'[2] and told me it was for growing illness in boys, and that I had to give the boy three fingers everyday of that medicine until it was all gone. I did, and it worked too. . . . I don't know what it was made of but it was a white creamy liquid."

"Well for me," Shae added, "I would never go to no hospital to have a baby. I had all my babies at home with no problem. My mother delivered her own babies. You know they used to keep you in there (hospital) so long after you had the baby. . . . You know you suppose to take the nipple (naval) string after it fall off and give it to the husband and let him bury it under the steps, or someplace where people don't walk," Shae continued. "If you bury where people walk, harm will come to the baby. I know some ladies who say if the nipple string fall off before they leave the hospital, they (hospital personnel) wouldn't give it to them. . . . I don't know if doctors (mainstream) know about colic. He'll (mainstream doctors) give you some medicine and tell

you your child got ear ache or something like that. And he don't, (have that) but treaters
know," Shae concluded.

Bae Bae and Shae[3] are both African-American women whose experiences
reflect the sentiments they and other members of the community have toward
traditional and mainstream medicine. This dialogue also illustrates how the
quality of health care in this rural African-American community suffers when
a person's folkways, values, and attitudes toward illness and disease are not
taken into account. This chapter focuses on the historical events that shaped
the dilemmas of health care in this rural African-American community—(1)
how the ethnomedical beliefs and practices came about, (2) how they survived,
and (3) how they were passed on.

Although it was many generations ago when the ancestors of Bae Bae, Shae,
and other African-American community members came to these shores, stories
about why they came, how they came, and in particular the pain, suffering,
disease, and dying that accompanied them are not forgotten. They remember
from the stories that were told to them by old grandparents and great grandparents—some of whom were ex-slaves. Others may not have been slaves, but
they witnessed the conditions or heard the lifelike tales of those slavery days
and hard times.

In the late afternoons and early evenings after emancipation, the front porch
served as the stage for family storytelling, similar to the ones so vividly artic-
ulated by the interviewees in this study. Persons from rural backgrounds
shared stories with me about the "old days." Storytelling is a routine practice
for them. As a result, family narratives were a very significant part of gathering
data on secret doctoring.

Many of the narratives about health care echoed feelings about mistrust
toward mainstream caregivers. To be enslaved, stricken with illness, and mistrust those who provide for your infirmity care can be a most unwelcome and
desperate situation. Distrust of mainstream medical establishment has not
been totally eradicated. According to Dr. Harold Freeman, Chief of Surgery
at the Harlem Hospital Center, a major "contributor to the ill health that
plagues our (Black) people is the strong distrust we (they) have of . . . the
medical establishment. . . . This kind of anger at and distrust of the medical
establishment can cause us (African Americans) to avoid all types of health
care—from preventive services to treatment of a serious problem" (Freeman
and Villarosa 1991, 60).

Health situations for enslaved Africans did not improve after liberation; as
a matter of fact they worsened during the post-emancipation era. As a result
of faith, determination, and the will to survive, the self reliance, which was
brought from West Africa, remained a part of enslaved Africans' cultural and
medical tradition. Africans taken from their homeland found themselves
thrown into a new and strange environment. This new environment was indeed a challenge and set the stage for many triumphs and tragedies. They had

to adapt the medical knowledge they brought with them to fit the new environment and the new social situation. Knowledge about new herbs had to be learned. Religious concepts had to be modified. Part of the beauty and strength of this area's rural African-American cultural tradition is the survival of this ethnomedical tradition that is thousands of years old.

Early African-American medical views were not so unlike early forms of folk Christianity, nor did they differ greatly from Native American medico-religious practices. In examining African-American ethnomedical practices, we must take into account the historical events which shaped the African-American experience. Consideration must be given to the consequences of the legacy of the African's belief in the supernatural, conversion to Christianity, and cultural mixing between Native-American Indians and Africans for example. In rural French Louisiana an African-American tradition survives among a people who have practiced, without questioning, this tradition from generation to generation. In many cases these practitioners offer very little explanation for their rituals. They practice to keep alive a custom because their parents, grandparents, and great-grandparents did so. They continue the tradition by exercising their knowledge about supernatural powers and because "it works."

Africans brought with them, as part of their value system, respect for elders. This custom continued in the Americas. Hence, it is taboo for young people to ask older persons questions in this society. You simply did not question your elders, to do so would be disrespectful. You were taught that learning was done by observation. Therefore, young people in this community are taught to value authority and age. Elders are viewed as superiors in wisdom and knowledge and as authorities in a proven way of life that is good for personal growth and development.

MEDICINE DURING SLAVERY

There is no known comprehensive study on the early medical treatment administered to enslaved Africans. Many early studies do confirm however that enslaved Africans were thought to be a strange species with their own peculiar kinds of behavior and diseases—distinctively different from Whites (Jordan 1950). Even though there is recorded concern expressed by slaveholders for the wellbeing of their slaves, for the most part the health condition of enslaved Africans was of economic concern for plantation owners. Trained doctors in rural Louisiana and other rural areas of the South were scarce, and most persons, Black, Red, or White, who needed medical attention relied on family knowledge about traditional forms of health care.

Although health care was provided for enslaved Africans, treatments were in most cases administered by plantation owners themselves, their wives, or overseers. Many of these people had no previous knowledge or experience with disease and sickness. They learned about medicine and practiced "physicking" according to knowledge they acquired from popular manuals of the time and medical advertisements in newspapers about various remedies (Darst 1971). In many cases knowledge acquired about certain cures for specific illnesses was obtained from their African slaves, who European Americans depended on to take care of fellow slave laborers. Nonetheless this physicking often contributed to the death of many enslaved Africans (Postell 1951).

Early African-American secret doctors utilized their knowledge of herbal remedies in dealing with ailments. These remedies were based on the cause of the illness—be it natural or unnatural. Often medical ethics and basic philosophy of western medicine clashed with that of Africans' whose beliefs were based on the supernatural. Early enslaved Africans were often required, in some cases against their will, to receive the treatments of White doctors. In spite of forced treatments, enslaved Africans maintained their own Afrocentric beliefs and practices associated with certain ailments, and they continued to engage the services of secret doctors. Secret doctors hid their knowledge about medicine, they administered their own remedies (which included herbal medications and/or amulets), and carried out other healing rituals behind closed doors (Savitt 1978).

During the plantation time, trained White medical practitioners were in competition with African folk doctors whose medical knowledge was based on information orally transmitted from generation to generation. White Southerners developed an exclusive branch of medicine for enslaved Africans, because they felt Africans were not of the same species as Whites. They were especially keen to bleeding and purging of Africans to cure them—a very painful treatment process (Gray 1979). The treatments administered, or approved, by plantation owners were frequently harsh and inhumane. These treatments coincided with slaveowners' beliefs that persons of African descent had a high tolerance for pain because they were less than human (due to the dark pigmentation of their skin). It is not surprising that this misconception was perpetuated throughout the era. The "ability to endure pain" is not a physiological one, but rather it is closely associated with the Africans' spirituality. Early religious convictions (prayers, sermons, spirituals) clearly show the Africans believed that if one "bears his/her cross," suffering brings joy in the end.

Perhaps the enslaved African developed a capacity to endure pain and suffering because they were in a situation where brutality, pain, and suffering had become a part of life; a life over which they had no control. The inability to endure would have meant deterioration and demise. Therefore, Africans viewed their new challenge of endurance as a means to hope, health, and everlasting life.

In contrast to the early popular belief that African Americans had a high tolerance for pain, Langley and Wolff (1968) cite several studies that suggest that African-Americans' tolerance for pain is less than that of European Americans, and that pigmentation plays no part in pain response. However, what is significant according to Langley and Wolff is that African Americans in the study did not complain (they bore the pain), versus the Europeans who complained. They further concluded that cultural attitude toward health and sickness, as well as one's religious attitude, influences one's perception of self; and these attitudes affect the way a person responds to pain.

Licensing of doctors in Louisiana began during Spanish rule in 1800 (Dart 1931). Physicians trained in western medicine began to arrive in significant numbers in about 1780 (DeVille 1973). One early document indicated that the early practice of medicine in Louisiana entailed three types of practitioners—surgeons, physicians, and pharmacists. Physicians could administer medicines internally, while surgeons were legally banned from this practice unless a physician was unable to be located. Certificates showing the passing of a medical examination and papers showing they were members of the Catholic faith were required documents to be carried by all medical practitioners (McMurtrie 1933). It was not until about 1892 that the State Board of Examiners was formed to regulate and grant certificates for the practice of medicine.[4] In 1882 the Opelousas region had thirty-one registered physicians, most of whom held diplomas from the University of Louisiana.[5]

Despite the many fatalities during the early stages of medicine, there were some successful contributions by early Louisiana doctors. Some of these doctors were of African descent. Du Pratz and Le Page, early explorers to Louisiana, learned the cure for yaws and scurvy, diseases common among enslaved Africans, from an early African-American folk doctor. Yet another enslaved African shared his knowledge with Cotton Mather about inoculation for smallpox; the vaccine was already in existence in Africa prior to the slave trade (Duffy 1958; Usner 1979).

In addition to the traditional forms of medicine practiced among early African Americans, records indicate that Blacks were formally trained as physicians as early as 1780. Some of those early doctors were located in Louisiana (Bergman 1969; Morais 1967). Traditional and trained doctors were both referred to as "doctors." However, what was important to the African was a successful cure rather than the title. As a result, many African-American folk doctors earned reputations as good doctors.

Black folk doctors treated both Blacks and Whites. Enslaved African's motives for treating Whites were often questioned. For instance, fear of being poisoned by African folk doctors was common among European Americans. These fears often were carried to the extent of court hearings to prove an enslaved African's guilt or innocence regarding health care of Whites (Porteous 1934). Thus, state laws were implemented to curtail the issuing of medicines by slave folk doctors, who had on occasions been called upon to treat their master's or the owner's family. If a fatality occurred, the slave doctor was often accused of deliberate intent. This is one factor which no doubt contributed to the maintenance of the secret tradition and the underground practice of making medicines. There was a continuing need to keep folk doc-

tors' identity secret—if you hid your knowledge about medicine, then you
were less likely to be called upon to treat Whites.

During the early Antebellum period enslaved Africans were often in the
forefront of treating and curing illnesses (Mitchell 1978; Laguerre 1987). They
were often sought after for their medical knowledge, which in most cases was
based on traditional forms of healing and preventing sickness. Early trust and
faith between African folk doctors and the African slave were strengthened
due to shared medicoreligious beliefs related to the causes of illness. Equally
important were the popularity and successes of the early African folk doctor
among both Blacks and Whites. Today there is growing interest in researching
traditional African healing practices.[6]

African-American medical knowledge was, and remains, a tradition based
on cultural nuances, despite its secrecy and the early formal training of some
of its members (Miller 1916). Even when some members achieved formal
education they returned, as they do today, to their respective African-American communities because there remains a preference and feeling of trust that
effective medical care can only be achieved through the services of one of
their own race. This is partly due to the racial superiority and lack of cultural
sensitivity often assumed by the mainstream medical profession toward their
Black patients. Herbs, ritual objects, prayer, and magic are universally applied
in healing rituals throughout the African diaspora. Folk doctors in the early
plantation era and today are respected, have spiritual reverence, and influence
the attitudes of people in the community.

Many early enslaved Africans who had superior medical knowledge and
success with treating, or who contributed to the cure of some illness or disease, were granted freedom and/or given an opportunity to acquire scientific
knowledge from a mainstream European physician. Elderly Black women in
particular were used by Blacks and Whites to serve as midwives, and much
of the midwifery tradition is credited to the knowledge of these Black women.

Jean Robinson (1979) presented an excellent study giving a historical account of the medical tradition of Blacks. She concluded that African Americans
having medical knowledge were effective and popular as health practitioners
in the colonial era. Contrary to popular belief, Africans during pre- and post-
emancipation did not leave their health care to chance. They were very health
conscious.

There are many pathetic stories involving medical discoveries as a result of
experimentation done on Black patients. The particular story about Cesarine,
however, advanced knowledge in the practice of obstetrics. Cesarine was a
mulatto child born to an African slave woman in 1831. She was named by Dr.
Francois Prevost, pioneer of the cesarean section, in honor of that successful
operation. Cesarine's mother was the first black woman on whom Dr. Prevost
performed this operation (Souchon 1915).

Self-taught European doctors did a lot of cutting, bleeding, opening of ab-
scesses, and amputations. Any form of cutting or surgery as such is still viewed

with skepticism among this rural African-American population. And it is often stated that "White doctors are too quick to cut on Black people." This form of treatment was quite foreign to the enslaved African and was not a part of the healing tradition of their ancestors. Or, perhaps surgery treatments could have been related to, or conflicted with, other cultural beliefs.

Evans-Pritchard (1937) observed that among East African people if after death one was suspected of possessing evil (sorcery or witchcraft powers), an autopsy was performed to locate the witchcraft substance. If located, the entire family of the dead person was determined to be evil and witches. Thus they became outcasts or suffered cruel punishment. Fear of treatments that involved cutting could mean fear of voodoo and curse (witchcraft/sorcery) accusations, since many illnesses among rural African Americans in the South are associated with unnatural causes like curse and hoo-doo.

This fear still persists today. The belief that "the white doctors don't mean no good" and that their intentions are mostly experimental are sentiments that are expressed among many African Americans. A prime example of Blacks being used for medical experimentation is the Tuskegee Project—a federal experiment on syphillis performed for over fifty years on several African-American men, without their informed consent, for the purpose of securing information on the long-term effects of the untreated disease. African Americans continue to experience similar discriminatory practices within the medical establishment, factors which not only continue to perpetuate feelings of mistrust, but also are contributing factors to other disease manifestation (Spencer 1993).

Failure to provide early medical treatment for slaves when they complained of illness is another reason Blacks were skeptical of the European-based medicine and treatments. Plantation medicine forced the survival of African-American folk medicine. The enslaved Africans brought with them their own medical system based on traditional African concepts about illness, health, and plant use. Because of the attitudes and mistrust toward white medical practices and the differences in cultural values enslaved Africans depended, to a great degree, on the traditional beliefs and practices that were a carryover from Africa, and to some degree, a diffusion with Native American culture. Their folk medicine tradition was not totally unlike other folk medical systems. In an article by Germain (1992), she asserts an estimated 70% to 90% of persons in the United States will first administer some form of self-care, or utilize the services of a folk practitioner, before resorting to mainstream medicine.

ORAL TRADITION

African-American folk medicine represents a purely oral tradition and is considered a legitimate form of ethnomedicine. Although it is not a written doctrine, it is a spoken creed that is remembered and passed down (Foster 1978; Vansina 1985). It is a carryover from West Africa, has existed since the beginning of slavery, and it continues to exist as an oral tradition today (Harvey 1981). Herbal and medical knowledge about what one does to avoid, prevent, treat, or cure a certain natural or unnatural illness is passed on orally within families from generation to generation. Like mainstream medicine, any new disease has to be coped with by trial and error until one finds the cure, and then the new cure is passed on orally.

Folk medical beliefs survived through oral narratives, sayings, and superstitious beliefs told in this rural community. These exist as a form of teaching to explain good and bad behavior; they also explain the concept of illness and its causes. Beliefs about disposal of hair, feminine hygiene, sin, disrespect, and improper dress are all examples of taboos that if not adhered to will cause illness and misfortune.

FOODWAYS

Food and nutrition contributed to and, in many cases, ruined the enslaved person's health. The enslaved Africans had very little choice in the selected diet they were to maintain. Some foods were eaten because of their health value, for example, yams. Other foods were eaten because Black slaves were concerned with survival and the desire to maintain at least a minimal state of health; so they ate what was available. The common meal consisted of pork, molasses, rice, and bread made from a corn base. These staples are still favored by many rural Louisiana African Americans.[7] Also available, but not in abundance, were vegetables; the yam or sweet potato, black eye peas, and okra, were the popular items in this category, and these items remain especially popular in this area.[8] These vegetables were grown by the slaves themselves when they had time to devote to gardens. Other food substances were periodically provided, but they were not a major part of the diet.

Eating habits were often aimed at survival rather than consciousness of nutrition. These habits carry over to present day. Pork consumption, one of the main dietary staples, is one of the leading causes of hypertension. Hypertension and heart disease remain the leading causes of death among Blacks. The slaves' diet was one that was acquired and was not representative of their African heritage. The early diets thus often resulted in diseases that were unfamiliar to the enslaved African and to folk doctors.

TERMINOLOGY

One of the questions this study raises is the use of language in relation to folk healing practices in Louisiana. This language, including terms such as witchcraft, and satanism, has misconstrued the meaning and distorted the image of Louisiana's folk healing practices (as in the case of Marie Leveau).[9] These ill-defined interpretations provoke uncomplimentary thoughts in readers' minds and portray African-American folk healing customs as bizarre and

irrational. Using a western paradigm for a folk-cultural concept has often resulted in the use of a language and analysis that is not representative of the
true cultural meaning of the folk healing (Kuna 1974–75).

There are several key definitions that are relevant to the clarification of the
function of all health systems. Seijas (1973, 544) defines a health system as "a
set of beliefs regarding the causes of illness and the ways in which illness is
handled and prevented." In addition health care systems are viewed as an
intimate part of the culture, because they are an extension of the community's
cultural values (Foster 1978). Beliefs about illness and disease in this community are intertwined with religious beliefs.

The African-American folk medical system presents a dilemma, because
while there is pride in the beliefs, there is confusion because of mainstream
medicine's attitude toward this aspect of Black culture. As one author states
"early literature often undermined the socio-cultural aspects of African traditional medicine. At times, these are reduced to ridicule simply because the
basis of traditional methods of healing is different in certain respects from that
of mainstream medicine" (Sofowora 1982, 119).

Terms often associated with this medical tradition, such as conjuring, hoodoo, voodoo, mojo, hexing, or witchcraft, are also a concern. These terms are
not applicable to the healing contexts of this research population. Misappli-
cation is the result of individuals who are usually outsiders writing about a
belief system that remains puzzling to them. Many terms and definitions have
been assigned to the practitioners. Some are accurate, some adequate, and
some simply misrepresent the tradition.

There are folk medicine specialists among the old secret doctors, just as
there are in Curanderismo in Mexican folk medicine, Santeria in Cuba, and
the healing arts in Haiti, Brazil, and West Africa (Watson 1984). In Louisiana
African-American folk medicine practitioners are all commonly called treaters,
or secret doctors, and in most cases describe what they do as secret doctoring
or treating. Most are considered general specialists. They treat most illness
and disease, natural and unnatural, physical and mental. Included among those
referred to as general specialists are Mr. Jacque who specializes in treating
snake bites and Miss Janey Bea who specializes in treating bone fractures and
sprains. Another type of specialist is one who treats problems associated with
mental health and is commonly referred to as a mind reader (ethnopsychiatrist). These practitioners are few. Then there is the "two headed" treater (a
person similar to a sorcerer or witch in other cultures), whose function is to
cause illness, or harm, to another via curse and voodoo rituals.[10]

Overall the traditional doctor is seen as central to the well-being of the
community he or she represents. The treater is accepted by community members as a legitimate healer of illness and disease with the power to manipulate
supernatural forces (Bacon 1973; Lancon 1986; Petterson 1963; Stewart 1971).

As I have previously stated, ethnomedical practitioners in this area define
themselves as "old secret doctors" or "treaters." For example, when I used

the term "folk medicine," it was irritating to early interviewees because they
did not understand what it meant; it may have been offensive too, because it
certainly didn't make it easy for people to talk to me. When I used the local
terminology, I had more success with interviews. I did not use the terms
hoodoo or conjuring, because in this culture those words mean evil. Rootwork
is another term that is not used because it also has vague meanings and implies
that one is "working" something on another person.

Feelings of reservation and mistrust were expressed to me by an interviewee, whom I will call Maran (which means Godmother), regarding local
medical practices and terms.[11] I was told by Maran that before I began my
research, I should make sure I didn't call the practice "traditional healing, or
nothing like that, cause that's not what it is. Call it what it is, 'Treatments.' "
As mild and safe as "traditional" sounds, it was still offensive to her, because
she like others in the community didn't know what it meant within the context
of what they believe. Treaters conceive of their practice as good. As one of
the treaters indicated to me "now what I do is the work of God, I don't
practice none of that other stuff." Most people who are insiders are defensive
about calling the medical practice any other word except the one familiar to
them. This is one of the reasons the practice remains hidden.

Another interviewee, who I will refer to as Auntie,[12] demonstrated a similar
response when I asked for information about "healing practices." She non-
chalantly sat in her rocker, pretending not to know what I was talking about;
then about a half hour later she said, "I don't believe in that foolishness." I
responded, "I certainly don't either! I just want to know about it." Convinced
that I had no other motive than wanting to know, she proceeded to get the
other members of her family involved in telling me two hours of narratives
related to old treating practices. Auntie's response is not uncommon. Nobody
practices, nobody believes, and nobody goes to visit treaters—yet they exist.

The rationale for this annoyance and avoidance of the terms herbalist, hoodoo,
conjuring, and other similar words are not because of negative connotations, but
because the secret doctors have fallen prey to stereotypical images of evil. In
truth their practices are spiritual; these connotations are some of the reasons why
folk healing in this community remains secret (Thompson 1984).

BASIC STRUCTURE OF MEDICAL SYSTEMS

The move to legitimize African-American folk medical practices can be
viewed as a movement contributing to the enhancement of the self-concept
and the reduction of stress/illness among Blacks. It is only when the medical
system of this African-American population is viewed within the broad context
of the total socio-cultural milieu that the health behavior and the validity of
the folk medical system can be understood.

There are five key structural similarities and differences of the folk medical
and mainstream medical systems. They are the concept of what health is, the

cause of illness, the treatments, the patient population, and the types of practitioners.

A Healthy Person

For the most part physical health is defined by mainstream medicine pathologically—a person free of germs or viruses based on clinical test results. Diagnosis is primarily of a mainstream scientific nature. People in this rural Louisiana community define illness culturally. A person who is unable to function in his or her role and becomes a threat to self and society is one who is considered unhealthy.

Causes of Illness

This community believes that there are natural and unnatural causes of illness. Natural causes are those ailments, for example, that are caused by dressing improperly and going out in inclement weather resulting in a common cold, flu, etc., and acts committed against nature. If someone has committed a sin or wrong against another individual (i.e., lie, theft, incest), then this type of natural cause is an act against God and the illness is based on the religious belief that God punishes.

The unnatural causes of illness are associated with intentional malevolent acts committed against another for the sole purpose of bringing physical harm or misfortune to the other. These malevolent acts are known as hoodoo and curse. Hoodoo (defined within this cultural context) is a practice that causes harm or misfortune to someone by using material elements, for example, poison herbs, hair strands, or clothing worn by the person one wishes to harm. A curse is to wish harm and/or misfortune on someone. It may be silent or verbal and is similar to the practices of witchcraft in other cultures (Middleton 1963). Folklore and anthropological scholars have used the terms magic (Frazer 1958), fetishism (Nassau 1904), conjuring (Puckett 1926), or rootwork (Hyatt 1973) to describe these practices in other cultures or communities.

Not all illness or misfortune is considered the result of curse/witchcraft or hoodoo/sorcery; rather those terms are usually used to describe those experiences that are the abnormal, profound, or unexplainable (Evans-Pritchard 1937, 70).

The Treatments

Preventing sickness is one of the measures taken by both mainstream and folk medical systems. For mainstream medicine, prevention is based on legal institutions and acts, such as the office of Public Health, quarantine, and compulsory immunization. Among this rural population, similar rural African-American populations (Snow 1977; Mitchell 1978), and West African communities (Conco 1972), preventive medicine is based on personal acts rather than legal institutions. Personal acts, committed by a person against another, are believed to be the causes of certain illnesses or the result of supernatural powers. So one must protect oneself from possible harm from others by employing the services of a folk practitioner. Therefore, for an illness that is a result of unnatural causes, amulets may be employed—material objects embodied with a divine spirit; in this case the protective powers of the Holy Spirit are usually employed along with other medicinals. Natural illnesses are thought to be caused by the forces of nature, and in most cases they are treated with herbs and other folk medicinals. Prayer is always employed for both natural and unnatural causes of illness.

The Patients

In this community the patients of the folk medical system are usually African American—males and females, children and adults—who believe in its efficacy. Many of the patients are local kinfolk or persons in the immediate community, although some secret doctors have patients in other places in Louisiana, the United States, Canada, Europe, and the Carribbean. These are usually relatives or immediate community members who have moved from the area. Because of the nature of the practice, it is important that the treated person has certain loyalties, trusts, and shared social and cultural traits. Secret doctors do not treat strangers; a stranger must be introduced to a secret doctor by a relative or immediate community member before he or she can be treated, and that relative or community member must also assure the secret doctor that the stranger can be trusted.

Patients cross class and racial lines. There are three major patient categories. First, there are persons who do not believe in modern medicine and prefer the old methods of treatment. Next, there are those who have not had success with modern medicine—consequently, they seek out other forms of cures or they return to traditional treating practices. The third category are those patients who use mainstream and folk medicine simultaneously. They are usually those who have some formal education, and they are not convinced that the old way is no longer effective. Some from this category also hold secret doctors in higher esteem and have more faith in their remedies. Some of these patients take the prescribed medicine of the mainstream doctor for a period of time, or not at all, and in some cases are likely to conclude that the mainstream doctor's medicine did not work. This partly has to do with unfamiliar prescribed treatments and the fear that the mainstream medication may do harm.

The patients of mainstream doctors are from both White and Black communities; however, if the mainstream doctor is White, then the majority of his/her patients are White. If the mainstream doctor is Black, then most of his/her patients are Black.

The Healers

Southwest Louisiana African-American folk medical practitioners today are described as "secret doctors, treaters, mind readers, and grannies." There is broad knowledge about herbal-lore among them. Healers learn their skill from someone in the family who is a secret doctor and who passes on the knowledge. Learning takes place at home, in some instances by observation. For the most part though, beginning secret doctors rely on themselves and call on a mature secret doctor for advise.

Experience, age, and sex play very important parts in determining the kinds of diseases and type of persons one can cure. Older male doctors seem to be able to cure severe illnesses in anyone of any age and sex. Female secret doctors for the most part treat children and minor illnesses in adults. This belief coincides with the community's loyalty and respect for male and female elders whose role in the community is the sharing of wisdom through experience.

In these case studies secret doctors are known as doctors of the mind, doctors of the body, and doctors of children and maternal care. Secret doctors treat most illnesses, but they do have their specialties. There are two folk doctor categories in this community, the old secret doctor/treater and the mind reader.[13] The treater works with patients who may have illnesses that are the result of natural or unnatural causes. Treaters are in many cases, elderly women and men who are called by the Holy Spirit to treat. The calling is similar to the spiritual calling African-American ministers of the Gospel experience. Secret doctors are affiliated with a Christian church. A person's credibility as a treater is recognized when he or she has successfully cured someone or is responsible for someone's good fortune by accurately diagnosing the illness. Diagnosis is usually based on the patient's complaint and/or complaints and observations from family members. It is not uncommon for an ill person to go to a secret doctor, a mind reader, as well as a mainstream doctor, in an effort to find relief.

Most secret doctors treat from the privacy of a bedroom in their homes. When being used, this space is off-limits to others, including immediate family members. The treating items of the secret doctors are always considered off-limits, even when not in use. None of the secret doctors utilize media advertisements, nor do they openly advertise by posting signs in front of their homes. They do not charge set fees for their services. Some suggest a price, saying: "a dime," "a dollar," or "whatever you have to offer." Others accept whatever the patient gives them, including in-kind donations, such as a bushel of okra, a crate of sweet potatoes, etc.

All of the secret doctors state that they are not opposed to mainstream medical practices. Nonetheless, they do not encourage it except in cases in which they feel their treatment is ineffective, and then mainstream medicine is recommended as a last resort for the health of the patient. The secret doctor is mainly responsible for treating and preventive medicine. He or she cures with herbs, other medicinals, and prayer. Amulets are also important for healing and preventive measures.

Mainstream doctors are usually White males and females (although some are Black) of various ages and class backgrounds. They have gone to academic institutions to obtain a formal education in medicine based on knowledge that is the result of scientific reasoning and is documented in writing. Hence most ground rules relating to practices and prescribed treatments have already been tried, proven, and documented as tenets. Also, economic gain is often the motivation for a career as a medical doctor. For secret doctors in rural Louisiana the charge is minimal, and the motivation is to be a servant of God.

Many studies have attempted to categorize the traditional doctors, however. Voodoo and hoodoo, for example, are terms identified with the practice but are considered by this community to be the negative aspects of folk medicine.[14] These terms are interchangeable and are borrowed by White treaters, which further complicates matters and contributes to the confusion about the ethnic origins of the secret doctoring tradition. Dorson (1964) asserts that borrowing from Black folk medical tradition exists among Cajun folk doctors. One way in which this borrowing takes place is by the use of the terms conjure and gris gris by Cajuns (persons of European descent). These terms, used to signify supernatural beliefs, are indigenous to the magico-medical practices of Africans and persons of African descent. Music is another instance where borrowing from Black culture took place in Cajun culture. According to Hodges (1972), African influences can be found in Cajun musical style and form. The reason for this (borrowing) is because both the African American and the Cajun American were socially oppressed by the dominant society, thus the cohabitation was on an equal basis. Another study[15] cites how misnomers have contributed to the confusion as to who assigns labels, and who is responsible for labeling in this folk medicine tradition—the researcher or the researched?

The topologies Baer (1982) proposes are good (I agree that ethnomedical practices among Blacks have been generalized and stereotyped); however, in trying to get a grasp on the body of knowledge related to the practice, I believe it is more important to understand why typecasting has often led to mislabeling. His typologies simply do not offer alternatives that would eradicate problematic terms and restore the validity of this tradition. None of his types gives the reader an indication that these secret doctors are indeed "doctors of medicine." The reader is left with the same stereotypical terms, leaving us to draw from memory bank definitions that are responsible for undermining a tradition.

It is important that we clarify the meaning of voodoo within the context of Louisiana. Can we, or should we, define voodoo according to the West African or Haitian concept? Is secret doctoring voodoo? The indigenous experiences of African Americans in Louisiana should be considered in attempting to understand a tradition that is based on an African, Native American, and French European heritage.

Voodoo (also vodun) is a religion with West African origin. However, voodoo in Louisiana no longer means the same thing as it means in West Africa or Haiti. According to Dunham, vodun is a "religion of Haiti based on African animism. Belief in an almighty god and a hierarchy of lesser gods. It is a word originating in Dahomey meaning god" (1983, 77). Hurston writes "Hoodoo, or Voodoo, . . . with all the intensity of a suppressed religion . . . has its thousands of secret adherents. It adapts itself like Christianity to its locale, reclaiming some of its borrowed characteristics to itself. Such as fire-worship as signified in the Christian church by the altar and the candles. And the belief in the power of water to sanctify as in baptism" (1970, 229). To cite Mbiti, "traditional religions are not universal . . . each religion is bound and limited to the people among whom it has evolved" (1970, 5).

But, in this rural community, the term or the word voodoo or hoodoo is no longer thought of as religious or benevolent. Perhaps because of the way it has been misconstrued from without and given malevolent meaning. In any case voodoo/hoodoo is now defined as nonreligious and harmful and is synonymous with practices in other cultures that are termed witchcraft, for example.

Concepts set forth by Evans-Pritchard and John Middleton are important as illustrative examples of the worldview of this rural population in reference to good and evil, rules related to social behavior, and illness resulting as a consequence of sorcery and witchcraft. According to Middleton sorcery is a means of social control, and religion exists to reduce or resolve social tensions and conflict. Evans-Pritchard, on the other hand, theorize that witchcraft is interrelated with all aspects of society and it functions to regulate or maintain social relations. I believe we can use these terms in the same way to apply to my data. Curse in this community has a parallel meaning to Middleton's definition of sorcery. And voodoo/hoodoo has a similar meaning to Evans-Pritchard's definition of witchcraft.

The magical practices of curse/witchcraft and voodoo/sorcery are very often reasons given by the secret doctors and mind reader as the cause of illness and misfortune. Beliefs that illness and misfortune are caused by sin (taboos), curses/witchcraft, or hoodoo/sorcery are common in this society, but not all people believe in this philosophy. Not all illness or misfortune, however, is considered the result of curse/witchcraft or hoodoo/sorcery; rather, it is usually those experiences that are the abnormal, profound, or unexplainable (Evans-Pritchard 1937, 70).

There are many causes of sickness, misfortune, and death. Many people in the community believe that curse/witchcraft and hoodoo/sorcery practices are done to them by persons who are envious or jealous. The most common motive given for a person who brings harm to another is a consequence of his or her envy and jealousies. Persons in this community believe that usually a person who tries to bring harm to another is a person who wishes to enter a higher social class or someone who desires to control and gain power over another emotionally. Curse/witchcraft and hoodoo/sorcery are basically confined to the immediate general community, and it is implemented by persons from various social classes. A person of a lower social class, for example, can have a person from a higher social class "fixed" (means the same as hoodoo). Normally, one does not retaliate with another hoodoo or curse action; but, rather one seeks the removal of the fix, and seeks divine protection from future attacks via religion—prayer, protective amulets, herbs, etc.

Hoodoo/sorcery is a magical ritual which involves the use of material elements, for example, personal belongings (hair, clothing, etc.) of the individual to be affected. Similar practices exist in studies done by Middleton and Winter (1963, 262) and Evans-Pritchard (1937, 38). A Curse/witchcraft act is accomplished verbally by simply wishing harm or misfortune to another individual or that individual's family members, such as a spouse or children. A two-headed person may be employed to carry out either one of these acts. Hoodoo/sorcery is believed to be the more detrimental of the two evils.

Generally, suspicion about these evil practices occurs among individuals of different family clans within the immediate community. Blood relatives, normally, are not suspected of employing curse/witchcraft or hoodoo/sorcery to other blood relatives. It is believed that close kin ties are from the same forces, so to make such an attempt is in essence attempting to harm one's self. Not that jealousies don't exist among relatives; it just seems that those feelings are repressed and interactions are avoided. However, it is not uncommon for the community to say that a husband fixed a wife or a wife fixed a husband. A possible explanation for this exception to the rule is that the husband and wife are bound by law and not by blood.

Children are usually not the targets of suspicion. If, in fact, there is suspicion between parent and child or between siblings, for example, then it is believed that the blood relative is not the person causing the harm or misfortune; rather, that person is being used as a vehicle by someone else outside the family clan.

The case that follows was given by a secret doctor as an example of curse/witchcraft. For several years a family had a series of illnesses and sudden misfortunes. They believed they were victims of curse/witchcraft. It is believed that curse/witchcraft acts can last for several generations, and that if a person denies a wrong or refuses to confess a sin before his or her death then illness and misfortune are passed on to the children. This continues until an individual in the victimized family line recognizes the constant turmoil and thus seeks the advice or services of a mind reader first and a treater later. In many cases, the fix is removed and order returns. Typically, besides the use of magic rituals, the remedy involves advising a person(s) to reunite with the institutional church, or honor a call to the ministry, or a call to the healing (secret doctor) profession. This is an instance where curse—in Evans-Pritchard's term, witchcraft—is another way of explaining the unexplainable.

The next example, cited by Tee Nom, another secret doctor, falls within the framework of what Middleton terms the dissociation process of "social conflict." Social tension develops when one suspects another. A young man from a middle-class farm family fell in love with a girl whose family were tenant farmers. The boy's family strongly disapproved of this relationship and was unable to convince the young man to end the relationship. Despite the strong disapproval by his family, the boy married the undesirable girl. At this point, the boy's family suspected the girl or her family of hoodoo/sorcery.

This competing to win the sympathy of the boy by both families is the central focus of the social relations and is also a part of the tension phase. When the boy married the undesirable girl, open accusations were made that the boy had become a victim of hoodoo/sorcery. This phase, open accusation, is the conflict stage according to Middleton and Winter (1963, 17). This phase is an attempt to rupture or revise the newly formed social relationship. The initial unreasonableness and sudden unexplainable behavior and decision of the middle-class boy to wed a lower-class girl is a violation of the social norm; hence, it has no logical frame of reference for this family. Therefore, they concluded that hoodoo/sorcery was the cause, and the person(s) responsible was the girl or her family. If we look at this in Middleton's terms, we see that this is another way of resolving social tension by giving it a name—hoodoo/sorcery—and a series of events. This type of disobedient behavior on the part of the offender (the boy) is believed to be a sin, an action that destroys the family unit (Middleton and Winter 1963). These instances are not merely an opportunity for a secret doctor or mind reader to help heal a physical or mental ailment, but are also a way of unfixing a bad (stressful) situation and making it good.

Overall, in addition to physiological causes, most illness seems to be associated with social conflicts and major life decisions that are chiefly related to social, health, and economic endeavors. To understand these practices in a broader reference is to understand how these religious medical practices function in this society as a means of regulating social behavior. Through the healing practices, these social conflicts are minimized; otherwise, social conflicts might result in chaos. In these small rural communities, one would expect to find cases, as in Africa, where social pressures are reduced through prayer and the healing beliefs of the practitioners. However, this does not negate the real understanding of the secret doctors and mind reader, that is, that their practice is purely religious and medical, and they do take away illness and disease.

One of the key functions of these secret doctors is their role as a special servant of God and hence their ability to bridge the gap between good and evil. A basic belief of the healing prophets in Soweto, South Africa (a similar belief exists among secret doctors) is that because their powers come from

God, they are stronger than those who practice evil; thus healing is more successful than affliction (West 1975, 103). West's remarks regarding his Soweto study further exemplify the role and function of healing in my study. He writes:

It is important that the prophets should understand why the illness has occurred, because this aspect cannot be separated from the cure. To cure one must understand what has happened and to understand what has happened one must know the why and the how. The prophet is concerned with the complaint and if necessary its whole social context. This reintegration function of the healer . . . is of great importance. Through the diagnosis the unknown becomes known and fear is often replaced by understanding. Thus satisfaction can come about only . . . if the world views of healer and patient in some measure coincide. (1975, 122)

Secret doctoring is a tradition that includes aspects of the old and the new. It is a Louisiana folk medical system that has been redefined and ill-defined without consideration for theological concepts. When Africans arrived in the New World they adapted certain principles and incorporated certain techniques into secret doctoring to deify its true character and more importantly to assure its survival. Secret doctoring became a syncretic tradition, one based on the integration of several cultural traditions (Bastide 1971). This folk medico-religious tradition is perhaps the most misunderstood aspect of Louisiana's African-American culture. Secret doctoring is complex, and an insider, such as myself, has not been able to fully penetrate it. It is almost impossible to paint a complete picture unless one becomes a secret doctor themselves, or if one betrays the sacred code of ethics. Then if this happens, a person risks the penalty of guilt—paranoia and community rejection. Usually a person who freely discusses the tradition with others (outsiders or insiders) is said to be a fake or that his or her treatments are weak.

SECRET DOCTORING IN THE NORTH

When southern African Americans began to move north, they took with them their medical beliefs and practices. The north offered limited resources to practice in traditional ways. Candle shops flourished and replaced the traditional home-based secret doctor. Candles, herbs, and home remedies prevailed. In many places such as the San Francisco Bay area, New Orleans, Miami, and New York contact with persons of African descent from the Carribbean, South America, and Cuba, influenced certain practices. High John the Conqueror became Shango, or was reidentified as Shango. Single candles and candles enclosed in glass with various colors signifying various West African deities were now being purchased to use on home altars. And in more commercial situations, the tradition became commercialized—people sought out these shops for malevolent as well as benevolent purposes (Wimbs 1989).

NOTES

1. Another common name for secret doctors (folk practitioners).

2. Teezon is a local name for a particular medicine. Its contents remain secret.

3. This dialogue is taken from one of the interviews I conducted in December 1988. Bae Bae and Shae are pseudonyms. Bae Bae is a widow, about thirty-five years old, the mother of a fourteen-year-old boy, with two years of college education. Shae is the mother of seven, and she has a high school education. She is married and is approximately forty years old. Both of the women have lived within the general vicinity of this rural area all of their lives.

4. "An Act to Regulate the Practice of Medicine and to Create a State Board of Examiners in Louisiana." Louisiana Statutes 99-101-103 (1892).

5. Registration of Physicians, State of Louisiana Under Act 31 of 1882. Reprinted from *Report of Board of Health State of Louisiana for 1882* (New Orleans: E. A. Brandao and Company Printers, 1883).

6. One such research project is being conducted by Drs. Charles S. Finch III, of Morehouse School of Medicine, and Robert R. Franklin, with Tulane University School of Medicine. See an article by Jeanie Stokes, "Traditional Medicine: More Than a Cure," *Tulane Medicine* 24, 1 (1993): 8–11.

7. Some favorite traditional foods are corn bread, coush coush (made from corn meal), cornmeal flap jacks (pancakes), molasses sweet bread, hog head cheese (a kind of meat loaf, made with the ingredients of the hog's head), hog crackling, and boudin (a sausage skin stuffed with rice dressing—a rice dish made with rice and chicken, pork, or calf liver, in most cases. Sometimes ground pork meat is used).

8. Some of the favorite local vegetables—the yam/sweet potato, okra, and black-eyed peas—originated in West Africa. See Chapter 8 for further discussion.

9. Healing rituals in Louisiana are usually associated with the ill-defined ritual practices of voodoo queen Marie Leveau and the supposedly wild orgies and sacrificial rites she held on the bayous. Voodoo was openly practiced by Leveau and others in the 1800s as a legitimate form of religion and medicine. It was at its height around the mid-nineteenth century. In the late 1800s, due to harassment by local authorities, the voodoo practice went underground.

10. I do not discuss the character nor the practices of a two-headed person (a person who is believed to possess supernatural powers, but who misuses that power to bring illness, harm, or misfortune to another), because I was unable to secure any significant data related to this type of practitioner. Furthermore, since this is an aspect of the tradition that is very much frowned upon, I did not want to confuse the issue by discussing both types of practitioners together. This mixing the good with the bad would have caused dissatisfaction among the population of my study.

11. Interview with Maran, August 3, 1988, Opelousas, Louisiana.

12. Interview with Auntie, August 6, 1988, Opelousas, Louisiana.

13. The mind reader is an ethnopsychiatrist. This study is primarily concerned with old secret doctors/treaters who treat physical illness, rather than illness associated with the mind. For a detailed analysis of the mind reader, see Wonda Lee Fontenot, "Madame Neau: The Practice of Ethno-Psychiatry in Rural Louisiana," in *Wings of Gauze: Women of Color and the Experience of Health and Illness*, edited by Susan E. Cayleff and Barbara Bair, Detroit: Wayne State University, 1993.

14. Voodoo in native terms is used to describe the work of the devil/satan. Hoodoo on the other hand is referred to as an act that is committed against another. You will more than likely hear the terms used for example as: "I don't belief in Voodoo, or "John hoodooed Mary."

15. "Traiteurs." Research project Number 91, Folklore Collection Archives, University of Southwestern Louisiana, Lafayette, 1968.

3

Secret Doctors Tell Their Stories

This chapter introduces individual secret doctors and their life stories. Some secret doctors weave very intricate and open tales, while others are more closed. The transcriptions are in the speaker's vernacular, and editing for clarity and space considerations have been limited.

Through these narratives we are made aware of similarities among the secret doctors that are representative of a cultural norm. Nonetheless, these personal narratives are their responses to social ills, discrimination, and unyielding adherence to their own healing tradition. Further, they represent what they feel is important. In addition they define their role as one of treaters, thereby providing insight into how they view their healing powers and why they continue to practice.

The following nine narratives consist of dialogue from three women and six men who practice secret doctoring, midwifery, and ethnopsychiatry. Secret doctors range in age from thirty-six to eighty-eight. Some have no formal schooling at all, or only an elementary education, while others are high school graduates. Two are the parents of college graduates. All are from rural farm backgrounds and have African ancestry; some also have Native American Indian heritage. A few have French family lineage, and one has Spanish ancestry. To protect the identity of my interviewees, I have assigned them pseudonyms. While these aliases are common to the area, they are not the ones for the individuals interviewed. These nicknames are used in the community to express kinship, affection, and familiarity.

TEE BEGBE

I was told about Tee Begbe by one of his patients. I went to see him in the small rural town where he lives. Upon arriving at his home, I entered from a side porch to the den/waiting room at the rear of his house where the sound of voices escaped through the doors. Six adults and one child were waiting their turn to be seen by Tee Begbe. "Como se va?" I asked as I entered and took a seat among the waiting patients. Some responded with "bon" or "pal mal" while others focused on me, a stranger. I knew the procedure. Take a seat and wait your turn. So I waited, my eyes examining the modest room typical of rural town working-class persons. Cloth covers concealed the torn or soiled spots on the aged sofa. Placed in different locations throughout the room were straight back chairs of the 1940s, darkened and browned from the natural oil of the many hands which contributed to their wear and handling of years.

As my gaze moved across the room, I noticed several pictures of Catholic saints, framed and unframed, tacked on walls and in corners. The experience for me was not new. As a child, and now as a researcher, this was a scene I witnessed in many homes.

The sound of the soap opera on the television made it difficult to hear the conversations taking place between the waiting patients—all Black, young and old. They were chatting, some in Creole French and others in English and French. I interrupted the conversation of one and inquired about Tee Begbe, who I was told was seeing a patient in the adjoining bedroom. A few moments later the door of the bedroom opened and a male patient exited. He was followed by Tee Begbe who glanced around the room and in French acknowledged newcomers, such as myself. He was a tall man, about six feet one inch, weighing about 190 pounds, seemingly of pure African descent. He had a slight bend in his shoulders, and he held an unusual walking cane. The next patient and all those before me were directed to the bedroom. When my turn arrived I went into the bedroom where there were additional pictures of saints and a crucifix. The room was quite orderly with two chairs near the bed facing each other. Tee Begbe motioned for me to take a seat in the patient's chair. I did. I told Tee Begbe who I was and who told me about him. "Vous parle Francis?" he asked. "Non, je pa un peu, peu francis," I responded. "Je non esh parle pa englise," he responded. In any case we managed to understand each other, and I concluded he was simply not interested in talking to me, especially in English. He further advised that I should come back when his son, who was working, could be present with him. I then asked if I could be treated for back pains, hoping this would relax Tee Begbe. He asked me a few questions in broken English and performed, I suppose, what was his usual prayer ritual. I asked if there was a charge and he said no, but if I wanted to give something that was okay. I went into my purse and pulled out a dollar in my fist. He motioned for me to put it on the bed. I did, and he covered it with the handkerchief with which he had been periodically wiping his face. I left his home with his blessings.

Later, I again contacted the patient who referred me to him. This time we went together to see Tee Begbe and his son was with him. Tee Begbe had no patients waiting, so this was a great opportunity for the second interview. After the usual introduction and purpose of our visit (the patient told Tee Begbe and his son about me, my work, and my purpose), the interview began in both Creole French and English. The patient who brought me there remained silent.

The following is a portion of the dialogue between Tee Begbe, his son, and me, and a third meeting I had with Tee Begbe alone. In revealing this dialogue, I am interested in the basic folk philosophy about health and medicine rather than the actual healing rituals, because they are considered sacred, and I was asked not to reveal certain aspects about them. Tee Begbe asked his son to conduct the interview with me, but he was present; and when he felt it necessary to say something, he did, and I indicate this by identifying him when he speaks.

"Things was so bad you couldn't hardly afford t'him (doctors). So God worked in mysterious way and showed somebody how to treat. And he treat for different thing that just a gift from God. And he (Tee Begbe) ain't got no education. He can't read and write. Just a gift he had it from God. I tell you what. Since I know myself he been treating. I am fifty-three and my oldest sister is sixty-four, and he start treating when he was young.

He is eighty-seven years old. He get around. He had never been sick a day in his life till he was about sixty-five. Then he had to have an operation. His old eyes. He had surgery for his cataract on his eyes.

He treat not just people but animals too. He was like a veterinarian. Now since he done got that age, he don't go out no more. He done give that up. Everybody come to him.

He started (treating) when he was twenty years old. Like a dream. God just told him what to do."

Tee Begbe: "My daddy treat and my grandpa treat."

"His brother was treating and was 106 when he died. His grandfather was treating all his life, and his grandfather the same. So that's better than two hundred years.

He treats for a whole bunch of things. I can't tell you everything. He treats for all kind of things, worms, baby ailment. He use the string for arthritis. He take three strings of thread, and pray on it and tie knots on them, and tie them on the part (of body) sick.

For the baby, sassafras tea. For women it's a certain kinda tea, it smell good too. For women Baume tea. That's just the French name, just the baume. Like a boy get a certain age that age bother you. He find a tea to make, and drink a gallon of that then you (boy) alright.

It's made from different trees. I know the roots but I don't know the name of the tree. I go get them for him. I can't go with you. No. It gon to be in the woods. If you don't know you can not get no root cause you don't know (knowledge about certain plants used in medicines is reserved for treaters only)."

Researcher: "I like that walking stick."

"That walking stick was made from a root that come from in the woods. They call that a blackjack. So see that wrapped around but you got to know what to cut in certain places (walking cane carved in curved and wrapped way as if snake wrapped around a branch). It's like for protection (can also serve amuletic purposes). 'Cause you can make a tea with that vine.

He see babies and stuff. Sometime one behind the other. Some time they got to wait just like a doctor's office, and some days they don't come at all. Depend how they do (sick).

After he gonna treat you, by the next day, by the night, you should feel better. It might hurt you more, but when that hurt coming to leave, it gon hurt you. But when that hurt is leaving you he know, because it gon hit him. He can treat you when it really hurting but you gonna be release because it gonna hit him for a while. It leave you, come through him, then it leave. When he use to put the string after two, three days that string drop and you feeling better when you look for it, then its gone. Then you don't look for it after it leave. Because it (hurt, pain, disease) leave with the string.

We trying to decide who is gon to be (secret doctor) between me and my baby sister. My oldest brother don't want it. We trying to keep it in the family as long as we can.

Close kin (secret doctors) don't do no good. We use to have a bunch old treaters but they almost all gone. So we would go see them and let someone else come here (not kin). Now we don't have much choice so we come here (to Daddy) for treatment.

We would bring them (children) to the (mainstream) doctor. But the doctor know certain things but they don't know all (what cause illness). My children have confidence in the treatment but they still young and don't know the responsibility of it.

You have to be kinda secretly when you treating. Like treating the baby with prayer. You have to be sincere. Not just any kinda way. You have to pray a certain way. For certain things there is different prayers.

Well, he say the prayers in French. That's how he always did say his prayers. He gon treat and say different thing, then I don't know. That's (prayer) kinda like the Holy Mary. It's a Catholic prayer. He Baptist. But that's how the prayer go. It's a prayer that was just passed on with certain treatment. Passed on, and when he started treating God showed him what he had to say. I can't say it unless God give it to me. It's secret."

Tee Begbe: "But you can say the (any) prayer you know. Any prayer is the same prayer. The prayer you know is the prayer you say."

"God got to call you out and show you things before you can be like a minister. Them education minister don't last long. Cause, I can say I preach! God didn't give it (skills and knowledge) all to me. Some thing I can do some thing I can't do. You see I told him as long as he would be able and get around I wasn't gonna stop him from treating. That's what keep him going. People keep coming and that's what keep him going."

NOC SOL

I was told about Noc Sol by his niece who, along with her parents, have gone to treaters all her life. Noc Sol mainly treats with prayer and herbal teas, salve, and poultices. When I arrived at his farm residence, he was out in the pasture cutting wood. Noc Sol's second wife of about twenty years greeted me, somewhat hesitantly, at the front door of their wood frame farmhouse. It was Fall, and she had the wood heater burning hot with oak wood. After the typical introduction, she suggested we walk to the pasture to meet Noc Sol. We strolled along the pecan tree-lined fence, stopping along the way picking and nibbling on pecans. Noc Sol was preoccupied, and he was not aware of our presence until we approached him. His wife explained who I was and my purpose. He was thrilled by the idea.

We all hopped in his old Ford pickup truck and headed for the house. He began to talk almost immediately about native medicinal plants, their uses, and how he acquired his knowledge. When we arrived, Noc Sol and I walked the pasture area nearer to the house, as well as the roadside, while he added flavor to the regional history of ethnobotanical plants with local legends and tales. He is best known in the community for his knowledge of herbs and their uses. Hence most of the data acquired about medical ethnobotany is taken from the lengthy interviews and plant samples given to me by him and another local medical ethnobotanist, Cousan Nom. Many of the medicinal plants were a part of his backyard landscape. He transplanted many plants since he uses herbs frequently.

"Oh it's (area) full of it (herbs) here. Take you tea for toothache. Get well two days. They (mainstream doctors) wasn't gonna pull that they (Blacks in olden days) pull that they self.

They got that sassafras, the white one, is for the little children for cold, or (corn) shuck tea. The red for the adult for the gallstone. Crook tea/twin leaves when children have a dry cough chest cold.

The carencro tea come out the swamp. That's for arthritis, stomach and healing the sore in the inside. That's how the Colored people, the runaway slave survive, with carencro tea. They haul dirt in the swamp made a big levee higher then that li'l house right there, and wide from here to the other fence yonder. And they stayed on that with they tea and corn and they made it till eh till the KKK would kill him and hung them.

You see my grandmother she was a secret doctor. She would send us, she'd give us a sack and send us go get some tea. And you had to bring what she want. She tell you what she want. Yea, and if you don't bring it, you go back again. My grandmother use to treat with tea. She was 105 when she die. People would come from all around. She boil and give so much per cup, make it strong, drink for two weeks.

People from Texas and from all over Louisiana call me for tea. Say how that's good!.

You take that (Carencro leaves) and put in your hat when you got a headache and it pull the heat out of your skull. That's (elderberry) very good for backache, inflammation, especially for women the root is white, boil the root. Carencro trees is male and female. They live a long time, been around for over 200 years. In 1882 the high water came and destroyed it. Now hard to find.

I am seventy-four years old, and she seventy-seven. My grand mamma learn it (to treat) from her mamma. That was Cherokee, them Indian from Monson, cross the Monson bridge going to the left that's all use to be their land. The KKK took that from them.

My daddy was Spanish and Indian. They (hospital) let him die. He was deaf and they let him die. He couldn't say what he wanted cause he didn't understand them. During, before the war it was bad for the Colored people. They had a war just for Colored. No White there. And him (his Dad) he was bright. They had him with the white and my brother went and seen him (in hospital). They find out he was colored so they threw him on the other side (Black ward of hospital). He was amongst the White.

About sixty years ago I use to pass to go get some baskets and they had some (Indians) along the road washing clothes in the ditch on they hand. They was still around about fifty or sixty years ago, some of them. Long white hair, way down here, white, white like snow. They find all kinda thing in the ground for them to eat. They get that for them to eat, root things to keep them alive.

The X vine for the growing up for the children when they reach twelve years old. The uncrossing vine to uncross your blood. You use the vine. Be sick you drink that. Some people be sick make bumps come out of you, but you get better. That's indian plant that there. For heart trouble, use pecan leaves.

The color of the tree tell you what kind of tree it is. Courtableu help reduce you, drink tea made from the bark. For those you use in the winter you use the bark and roots. Yea, I know a plenty herbs. Hard to find noddy."

GRANNY YA

The visits to Granny Ya were as if I was going back in history. She resided in a small wood frame double shotgun type house. Granny Ya's house was typical of the custom for the region, where space was of essence and funds were limited. The living room doubled as the main bedroom. Decoration was typical of years gone by. Family photos orderly placed, stiff white doilies decorated table tops, handmade quilts draped a four-post old fashioned bed, peeling linoleum protected the remains of the wood floors.

Several of Granny Ya's great nieces were departing her home just as I was arriving escorted by another great niece who had brought me there. The escort introduced me and asked Granny Ya's permission to be interviewed about "old ways of midwives and treating." Granny Ya remained seated in her ancient rocker which complimented the rest of the house ornaments. As I reached out to shake her hand, I could not help but notice the strength which marked her troublesome face of eighty-six years. She is arthritic. She wore a full apron, typical of the women of her generation. Once a full time midwife, Granny Ya works mainly as a folk doctor, treating children mainly for childhood illnesses.

"It's been so long (since I been treating). You see I was a midwife, and I been working on people, after I stop being midwife. (As a midwife) Well, I treat on them and place the baby for 'em. I never run my hand in 'em, but I just put my hand on them and I pass my hand on them (pregnant women).

Sometime the doctor said they had the breech baby. Sometime I'd turn them over and after I turn them over they had the baby alright. I done stop that (midwifery). I am full of arthritis. Let somebody else do it.

I tell them (pregnant women) to go to the health unit, that's where I take my course. On the first old Dr. Pateau, he the one give me my paper (certificate). I could go any where I wanted and deliver babies.

Sometime I'd call the doctor, sometime the doctor would call me. I was twenty-five when I started. I delivered until I was seventy-three. I delivered in a year, sometime about 100–200 babies.

I could tell if they would be having twins when I'd come there. So I call my son, 'come yer and help me.' Well, after the other one finish (is born), the other one (baby) put itself in its place.

I put a red rag around them when I think they gon miscarry, and it hold the baby there. When child got asthma, or got attache (overgrown liver), I put the red cloth on him and they okay. If they get sick again they put the cloth back on. (She used red strips of cloth for women of childbearing age.)

This is a gift from God. I am widow. I go to church every Sunday, and I ask the good Lord to help me with all their (patient's) trouble. I can tell what I do to a man but not to a lady. If I go to treat on a person it will not work (if she tell to a lady).

I am eighty-six years old. My mamma was a midwife. They had doctor in the old days. A white lady was having a baby once and had trouble. White Dr. Watt was there, but they call my mamma. She went in the kitchen and made a little sweeten water (gave to the baby). She (Granny Ya's mamma) say that baby gone live. That boy still alive. There were men midwife ... people just deliver baby, could be a sister or brother. In them time you didn't register no baby.

There are a heap of big children who speak to me say Grandma how you doing you the one help my mamma bring me in the world. One man say Grand Ma am not gonna leave my children call you Grand Ma. I am gonna have 'em call you nan nan. I say I don't care how they call me just don't call me too late to come to the table, ha ha ha! (Meaning don't forget to invite her to dinner).

In the olden days they (new born babies) had to have everything close and stay in there (house) nine days, and then they come outside and see the sun and the eye open. Now them baby come here. Time they come here they got they eye wide open like they want to talk to you.

You couldn't eat no arsh (Irish) potato, corn, fish, cornbread you could eat biscuit, or bread, some thing light (just after having a baby). Yea, I catched a many babies."

MISS JANEY BEA

It wasn't easy getting information from this family with a long history of secret doctors—both living and deceased. I was particularly interested in the older woman (the mother of Janey Bea) in this family, because she was highly regarded by family and community for her knowledge of herbs and treating. She acquired this knowledge from her American Indian grandmother. In any case, my first stop was Janey Bea's great uncle, also a secret doctor, who was about eighty-nine years old. He gave me a migration history of the family, as well as basic data on treating as he knew it. He then consistently and strongly urged me to pursue his niece (Janey Bea's mother). Any recommendation to see someone younger than they I interpreted to mean the younger person had extraordinary skills.

I went to see Janey Bea's mother, a sixty-five year old widow, at her home, which was about five miles from her uncle. On the first visit she was in the mist of preparing for her son's porch wedding. Porch weddings are another tradition that is slowly vanishing. We talked briefly, and she asked me to return for specifics. When I returned several days later, it had rained and I had a difficult time getting through the mud and water on the dirt road. But I made it, and Janey Bea's mother was waiting on the front porch for me. She is a very vibrant and active outdoors person of sixty-five, always tending her yard or garden. Although she was very warm, friendly, and giving of her time, she never entrusted me with any data until after several visits, and then that was limited. She was more interested in giving me the family genealogy in painstaking detail which was fascinating. Her strong Native American Indian ancestry is typical of many African-American families in this region. She did reveal, however, that much of what she knew about medicinal plants came from her Native American Indian grandmother.

On each of my return visits she did the same thing, proudly showed off her lovely family photos and told me parts of her family history. On one occasion I shared with her the local famous bone soup she had prepared, and on another she shared her knowledge about a few herbs. But she never talked about how she practiced, if she practiced at all, because she never admitted to being a secret doctor. Anyway, finally after seeing that I was sincere, she adamantly insisted that I talk to her daughter, who she said, knew a lot about herbs and treating.

As she requested I went to see her daughter Janey Bea. She was quite attractive and looked about thirty, although she was much older. She was in every sense of the word contemporary—jeans, soap operas, and the whole bit. She resided with her husband and three children ranging in age from sixteen through twenty-one. The home was very modern brick, indicating upper middle-class status. Her dress and appearance contributed to the status and revealed nothing traditional about her. It contrasted with that of other women in the community who were secret doctors like her—both young and old. This image I discovered was misleading, for in her thinking about secret doctoring, Janey Bea was just as traditional as all the other secret doctors.

Despite her denial that she practiced secret doctoring, she was basically cooperative and gave unselfishly of her time. She explained how she acquired the gift of secret doctoring and her basic religious philosophy connected with the tradition. She focused the initial conversation on her herbal knowledge, most of which was references to books and herbs found in the local health food store. She began by telling me about her experience with an illness that almost caused her death. This experience led her to seek out knowledge about herbs and cures and the desire to practice. Her experience resulted in her faithful and extensive use of herbs in the treatment of others.

"I had a dream about a old man telling me to use different herbs and mix them together and drink for a certain length of time. I have a herbal book that I use that tell me what things are good for. I don't use any doctors medicine. Doctors really don't believe in it (herbs).

After I got well (from her near death illness), this doctor saw me and ask what was I doing because I was looking so healthy and the only answer I give him was it's a blessing from God.

I learned about cream of tartar from an old guy. A lotta people don't believe in the old treatments but I do. I told him my stomach hurt all in the bottom and he told me that was probably my female organs and he told me to take cream of tartar and it was good for that (female problems) and he told me it was also good for people to get pregnant.

I use most herbs from the store and the peach leaves from the tree. Cause some of that stuff I might not know what it is and I might get a hold of the wrong thing. I don't want to poison myself and people. And the reason I don't use too much of those in the field because they poison (pesticide companies are hired by local farmers to spray their crops) a lot to kill insects. That's the reason I don't fool around with it too much.

Everything (native herbs) I could put my hand on before they started poisoning, I had it. People use to call me granny. You know like granny on the 'Beverly Hillbillies,' mixing up potions.

I don't treat, or nothing like that if they ask my opinion, I'll tell em. Healing has a lot to do with faith. Back in the olden days that's all they use was herbs and faith. My aunt use to treat with nine knots (on string) and nine prayers. She had a stroke and she passed it on to me. Some people who come I'll do it for them if they believe (in the string).

My daddy use to treat for sprain with the nine knots and nine prayers; it work for sprain. But doctors won't do you any good. And how it work for him he (her daddy) had a dream one night and said that was what he was to do. But he said 'not me I'm not good enough to do nothing like that,' and he left it alone. He fell and sprain his arm and got down and down. And so he started (treating) on himself. And went on and on. And before he died he pass that (knowledge about sprain treatments) to me. And a lotta people come for that (sprains).

It's a older man give me another one (treatment) and it go with nine again but no string is involved. But it's good for sprain and just about anything. I use my fingers and it's a prayer you say nine times. But the one who come must believe. The prayer it's not nothing superstition, voodoo or nothing, just prayer, plain prayer. You stop and you think and you read the Bible back then Jesus give people power to go out and heal people, and it was with prayers, and it's nothing but prayers.

This one guy really believe with all his heart, he fell off his horse and he came here on crutches, and he say I hate to worry you, but I come to see you I got to see you. I say it's about time you go to these (mainstream) doctors.

He say 'no I been they didn't do no good.' After a while after I treat on him he walked away without the crutches. The same thing happen to my daddy. It's really your faith your belief. Because I tell them I am not doing this it's Jesus, don't say I am good, I am not doing this 'cause it's not me it's Jesus, I am just doing it for him in his name.

And it really work and it work for myself. I would think, you know, before I really start believing, now how would a little string really help somebody out, and not thinking about the prayers on there and the one who said it in the name of Jesus. If you read the Bible a lot I get a lot of understanding about it, and about this herbal stuff. All before I was wondering, now I really believe it. I done seen it and my heart done conceive it.

Usually it's (prayer) kept secret not say secret, but you don't tell people what the prayers itself unless you pass it on to someone else. But it's plain prayers people use. I don't know why they say don't tell. It's the one who have it say they pass it on to somebody else and they tell like that. I don't know why they just told me to keep it to myself.

My daddy had cancer and he was dying and he wanted somebody in the family to have it but he wanted somebody to ask and they never did. So my husband told me why don't you ask your daddy. He was about to die and that was something good that he was doing and they won't have no more old treaters. So he (dad) told me then that what he had been wanted for me to ask him. And then my auntie after she had the stroke, she have children she has a bunch of children, but she didn't give it to her children she passed it on to me.

But what it started with, this old guy he was reading the Bible one day and I said what you reading let me see, and he showed me and we went into a discussion and he said it seem to me as if you have a lotta faith. He said I am getting old and sickly. Before I forget this is something good and I'd like to pass it on to you. And that particular day he told me what to do and I been using it.

I have people who just call, I don't know what difference, but you have to know their name, place they hurt and things like that, and it work too. When he, Daddy first give it to me, I didn't use it. I thought about it and I just put it out of my mind and I started saying like I didn't feel I was good enough, ready. And I know that I have sinned. My cousin sprained her foot. So we sitting here talking. So my husband say you know her daddy passed on the treatment to her. 'Well' she said, 'if you know what to do I don't care how ready you are, I am ready. I am going to be your guinea pig if you scared,' she said, 'go get a string whatever she need.' Two days later she wasn't on her crutches she was just hopping a little bit. It take a while. It don't just go away like black magic. But still at that I didn't go on from there. I said I going to wait a while. I said she forced me into it.

So one evening I was lying down. And I was thinking 'bout all the Lord has done for me. According to the doctors I am suppose to be dead. He must have spared me for some reason. It's five years. If he has done this much for me then I can do something to help the people. Nobody came for a time then this old lady ask my mom if my daddy passed it on to anybody. And she told her me. So the lady came here and look like it started coming to me. I wanted to do it. Things started happening in my life and my faith started building up more and more. And it just came to me I say God has to put something in your life to make you get up and start working for him.

I never ask why, but every treatment somebody ever give was always nine— prayers and things. Dr. Locks believes in this on the Wichita Road. The real older (mainstream) doctors believe in it because of their grandparents. I don't charge a penny, some people take charges for it. I been treating about ten or twelve years.

A lotta priest don't believe in this. My dad was Indian and lotta of it came from Indians cause they believe in that also, and Africa. But a lot of what Africans believe is voodoo (meaning evil, witchcraft, sorcery). It was just handed on from one generation to another and a lot of these Indians would treat these people that were sick didn't matter whether white, black, whatever. The Indians use a lotta herbs. I don't know how the string came about. My dad said it came to him in a vision.

The calling people deny or fight against it at first. When God call you to do something it's no running. I don't think it is as plentiful as it has been because a lotta of these young people they don't have time for stuff like that and the older people are dying and they not asking for it, or passing it down, or picking it up, or whatever to me. To my idea this is my opinion that its gonna come back strong as it has been cause people have really come to depend on it. That's my thinking. Because it's a lotta people now realizing that doctors now not really doing things for strain and stuff like that. A lotta young people are beginning to see that the doctor can't do anything for them like I had a young boy about thirteen or fourteen here the other day who really believe. His grandmother brought him. A lotta White people believe in this and they come to see me."

MR. AND MRS. JACQUE

The sun was a bright orange, seemingly almost touching the earth in some far-off distance, one late afternoon as I traveled down a winding dirt road in search of Mr. Jacque, whom I was told was a very fine old doctor. As I approached Mr. and Mrs. Jacque's homestead, I thought, is this America? How many have passed on the main highway and ignored this winding dirt road that seems to lead to nowhere. It was so isolated, peaceful, and remote. Sounds of nature were my only company. When I appeared on the doorsteps of their wood frame home, I had no idea of the treat I was in for. Several interviews were conducted with both Mr. and Mrs. Jacque. Mrs. Jacque, a very agreeable woman, did most of the talking, even though it is her husband that is the treater. He had some reservation about describing what he did and how, so his wife volunteered to do the talking for him. She described his practice in detail. Mr. Jacque was always present for these interviews. Only when he disagreed or felt something needed to be added did he offer his opinion. I was convinced that if he was doing the talking, he would say the same thing. Perhaps he was interview shy, or perhaps his apprehension was valid. Whatever the case, he approved of his wife sharing a wealth of information with me, while he basically oversaw the direction of the interview.

This was an unusual couple who looked much younger than their ages (they were both in their early sixties). They were homesteaders, as are many of my interviewees, and Mr. Jacque spends his time hunting, fishing, and doing a little farming. Mrs. Jacque was a victim of an illness that left her totally blind at the age of forty-three. That did not discourage her spirit, however. She learned another language, Braille, in a matter of a few weeks. She continued her hobby of flower gardening indoors. She also did various crafts, such as ceramics, that she proudly displayed throughout their home. Most encouraging was her sense of humor and zest for life. Mr. Jacque had just as much passion for life as his wife. Both were open and paternalistic toward me. This behavior helped me to ask follow-up questions I would not have normally asked, or would not have asked in detail. Mr. Jacque was also instrumental in sharing his knowledge with me, as well as samples, of home-prepared medicines. They also showed me how to make healing necklace amulets.

"I don't know if there is too much I can tell you cause there is not too much I know," began Mr. Jacque.

"On secret doctoring?" Mrs. Jacque asked and continued for the duration of the interviews. "This is an old historical place and it been around about over a hundred years or so. They had a lot of people who come over here with a lot of tradition. They came from Africa or Haiti. My grandmother came from Haiti, and it was not too much said about these people, or what they did because they believe in the signs (supernatural beliefs).

At that time they couldn't read or write, so they just did this (secret doctoring) in the small rural area. And a lotta people (White) didn't believe in this. How this come about is because of the church racial situation, and they (Blacks) couldn't exercise their gift that God had given them. So they were sort a like robbed of the lacking of wisdom and knowledge to (communicate with) the Holy Spirit. Now this (folk medicine) is coming back alive again, and people have more liberty to reimprovish (relearn) the power God has given them to use.

This old man (a next door farm neighbor) give this gift to my husband along with my prayers (she prayed for him to be blessed with the gift). So I can tell you, for him, how it (secret doctoring) goes. The old man would always bless the children (theirs) in Creole so they wouldn't get snake bite. Because of the swamps around here, picking cotton, blackberries, and in the old outside toilets, black widow spider hibernate in there and ground moccasins.

To get this secret (secret doctor knowledge) you had to know something about how to speak some of these words in Creole French. My husband was afraid to use it. He was not a believer (at first)."

Mr. Jacque interrupted, "I believe because I know it can be done and I saw it done. My bird dog had gotten bitten and she (next door farm neighbor's daughter) doctored on that dog. She use a string and the dog got better almost immediately. So that's when I became a believer."

Mrs. Jacque continued, "They tell me that you can't get the full strength of doctoring until about ten years. We don't want to have these kinda things lost. My grandfathers died at the age of ninety-one, and they believed in herbs and miracles."

Mr. Jacque: "You can't just pick it up, you got to go into it; you have to practice. If you got another person who practice and already know you can practice together. But if you practice in front of somebody that don't practice, they can take it from you, and that would weaken you. Part of this is because children or young people misuse this gift or play with it. You wouldn't give children something powerful like that to play with, unless they could be trustworthy and they would get a right age to inherit it. That's why they say it take that long to see how that child would mature and benefit, how much they would be obedient with that."

Mrs. Jacque: "You mixing faith healing with secret healing. You find this in Corinthians 12, gifts of the spirit. The nine knots is for the nine moons and nine months it take to make the baby born. The string is for the navel string, the line is the tree and the children is the branches. Now you have seven months for the seven angels, the books of Ezekiel, Verse 16, for the stopping of the blood. You can do evil with it as well as good. You can read all this through the Old Book of Prophets (Old Testament). And the book of James in the New Testaments, through study and practice you learn. A life of prayer must be lived. You suppose to believe in our culture and our heritage too. You suppose to make it prosper.

We have most of the things our people integrated from the old world and the third world and brought these things here. Our old ancestors talked, they lived it. They give you the words (Creole language and prayers in Creole); if you can learn the word then you got it. Chapter 16 in Ezekiel is a part of it. You can only get the word if you want the gift. You (a woman) can pass the word on but if you (she) pass to a woman it doesn't work, it weaken you (her). You have to want the gift first and the person has to want to give it to you and feel you have sincerity."

Mr. Jacque: "Number has to be uneven if you doctor with even it don't work. That's about all I can say."

MADAME COLOSSI

I never got a chance to meet Madame Colossi in person, although we talked briefly on the telephone. She passed away before we could arrange an agreeable meeting time. However I did meet with her daughter, an aspiring secret doctor, who was generous with information about her mother's philosophy on ethnomedical habits. When I arrived at her home, her daughter, daughter-in-law, granddaughter of two, and an elderly female cousin, who is also a knowledgeable midwife, eagerly greeted me. Thrilled by the idea of having someone come to interview them, they were a bit anxious.

They were proud people and they were not ashamed to admit they were believers as well as practitioners. We entered the small four room shanty house which housed several families (her daughter, her husband, and three children; her son, daughter-in-law and grandchild, and another son and his family). The extended family tradition was very much alive and visible here. When we entered the front room, which doubled as a living room and extra bedroom, I was immediately taken by the unusually enormous amount of saintly status and photos. Every wall and every corner was "protected" with one or more saints or crucifix. In one corner, high to the ceiling, was what I interpreted to be an altar. I inquired but I received a very evasive response. "We're Catholics and we believe in saints." In any case this subject seemed to be off-limits, so I didn't pursue the questioning about what was obviously an altar of some sort.

This family was bilingual, and Madame Colossi's daughter boasted that her grandparents were literate in "pure French." The interviewees spoke for the most part in Creole French to each other, and at times to me. The daughter-in-law occasionally confirmed what was being said and sometimes added to what was said. The older female cousin, of about seventy-five, did not participate in the interview. She sat in the rear of the room, and when Madame Colossi's daughter was unsure of something, she asked her elder cousin's opinion and approval in French. When she was satisfied that she was saying the right thing about her mother, or the medicine tradition, she proceeded with the conversation. From what I gathered Madame Colossi was an excellent treater who mainly concentrated on women and childrens' illness. She used two herbs, basil and mint (baume) tea faithfully, although she had knowledge of others.

"Mamma always kept this (basil), and we kept it up for childrens that come here, and that mint good for womens who just had a baby with a lotta cramps. Mamou the bark of the tree and the root good for cough syrup, and the seed good for a tea for chills, pneumonia, and bronchitis.

You don't bring them children to the doctor for no worms. Them doctor (mainstream doctors) don't know nothing bout that. They give some medicine and give some shot and that gone kill them. Take la pa sabb (worm grass), you boil till real green and made a syrup with it, and give the children with worm. Boil the flower for the inflammation. For women they boil like a tea then put in boiling water and sit over the pot, steam will pull infection out.

She picked herbs when they start to dry up, any time of year. During the winter time they dry up and you pick them, then store by putting in bag and hang up. The mint stay green year round though. The Indian lady taught her the prayers for treating. She never did tell me what her prayers was. She always did say her prayers in French to herself. If somebody ask, you not suppose to say. We didn't know (what the prayers were) cause we never did ask and you couldn't hear what she said. Just any prayer she said you had to pray. Prayers is the most important thing, more than anything else, prayers can do anything. She would always say a prayer. The only time you could tell somebody the prayer, like if a man wanted the treatment a lady could give a man the treatment but a lady couldn't give another lady. But if she was ready to let it go and not use it again, well then she could give it to a lady.

She could not read. So it was a prayer she learned. It is something that she could say from the heart. She just prayed over you. She put her hand over the part that was sick. Depends on what it was. For some (sickness) you had to come for nine days consistently, some every nine days, and some every three days depends on what it was.

The number nine is the same as a novena. You see for a novena you go (say them, or go to church) for nine days, and the prayers are suppose to work within nine days. So at the end of nine days you start another nine days.

She would treat anywhere in her living room. Anywhere you wanted to sit she start the treatment right there. Much of the treating knowledge has to do with just advising about various remedies. It didn't make a difference; the house would be full and she would treat. The house would be full from seven o'clock in the morning, six thirty people would be lined up, until night at nine, ten o'clock. People from all over come—Missouri, California.

Treatment last fifteen minutes or less. Some treatments had to be broken down in three different treatments. She'd treat for a few minutes, then wait, then treat, then wait, then treat again, arthritis for example.

Her mother also give (her) the gift along with the Indian lady. She was young, had just gotten married about forty-six or forty-nine years ago. The Indian lady from Elton just told her things one time and she caught on. She (mother) was raising a family and she didn't have time for it. After her family was grown she started using it more. She treated all colors of people. Some people still call for her. In a matter of speaking it is hard on a person to treat. Let me put it this way, she use to tell us if you don't treat the right way, it could fall on you (you could get sick with the illness trying to cure) whatever you treating for. So you got to know what you doing in order that it won't fall on you. You have to put your mind on that and nothing else. Because it is spiritual. That's exactly why a lotta young people don't treat!

You know like she say it was a time when she learned she had too many children to get right into it. She kept it up, but she really wouldn't do it unless she had to. Like if somebody would come that knew she did it (treat) then she would (treat), but other than that she didn't let nobody know she did this. She didn't advertise.

But on the end once she had started with one person and it kinda got out a lot. Well then everybody started coming, then that's all she would do. On the end she had to kinda tell them it was too many, cause you know it's kinda hard on a person, it's really hard.

She wasn't in no special frame of mind. She usually joke after she finish. She'd sit quiet and she would pray on you. After that go back to laugh and talk just like nothing going on. She did use strings, like for a lady that has an open back, after (giving birth) a baby, or (a damaged back from lifting a heavy object) lifted something too heavy. You know some womens they go three and four months without stopping from a period or something, well she would use a string and you would keep it on for nine days, or so many days until you lose the string.

Another thing she would use string for well like a lady would miscarriage, or threaten, you would keep the string until about a month before you suppose to have the baby. Depends on what it was for, the miscarriage it was a red thread. For the back open, any white thread, for the heart worms, a black thread. They always did that in the olden days they ain't had no doctors like they had today."

The following three biographies are on Secret doctors who basically did not permit a tape recorder, although I was allowed to take notes. What follows is a summary of those interviews.

BEEDEAU

Beedeau called himself a secret doctor. He had some secondary school education, was eighty-six years old with a younger second wife at the time of his death in 1989. He was Catholic and a retired farmer who, when not treating, spent most of his day fishing in his pond for catfish and perch. He treated for sixty-eight years and saw about five to six patients a week. He said that during the old days he used to see lots more. His treatments took anywhere from fifteen minutes to nine days. Beedeau referred to himself as a "secret doctor that treats." Beedeau also said that he received his gift to treat from God. As the father of eleven children, he said that his children were always ill and he couldn't afford to take them to a doctor, so he prayed for about a year asking God for the spiritual gifts to treat. One night around 4 A.M., while lying awake in bed, his "wish" was granted. He began treating his own children and was so successful that he began treating kin and others. Beedeau treated Blacks and Whites, males and females of all ages. He treated all kinds of illnesses in adults, for example, stomach ulcers, sores, arthritis, and chronic depression.

Prayer and the string amulets were the main elements Beedeau used to treat. In addition, he utilized an altar (most other treaters use their bedroom dressers or a table in the bedroom). This original altar holds photographs of former and current patients. Some of these photographs are thirty years old and include some of the more serious cases he successfully treated. One example of the more serious cases Beedeau pointed out to me, and the case he considers his most successful, was the photo of a man who was about to be committed to a mental institution by his family, but in a last attempt to help him they brought him to Beedeau for treatment. The family complained that the man was not motivated to work and he refused to socialize with others. He would sit and stare into space for days. Beedeau was successful in bringing the man "back to his right senses." The man is now a productive part of society, working successfully as a carpenter.

These photographs are not only evidence of Beedeau's success but they were also used in the healing ritual, and they are believed to give power to the altar. The altar appeared to be both functional and sacred.

TON GE GE

Ton Ge Ge is a male secret doctor who simply calls himself a "treater." Ton Ge Ge has some secondary school education, is about seventy-five years old, a Baptist deacon, and a retired farmer. He too is married and has several grown children. Although retired, he is still actively the chief administrator of his farm business affairs. Physically he is taller than average, about six feet. He has been treating since he was nine years old. Ton Ge Ge's first experience as a treater was when he healed a relative's horse of warts. Ton Ge Ge recently reduced the number of patients he sees from 12 to 10 a week. He says his gift to treat is a gift from God, and he was called by God to treat. He said for almost a year he continued to deny that calling, but the Holy Spirit would not let him rest until he accepted his calling. Before he accepted his gift, he had sleepless nights, sickness, and continued to hear the voice of the Holy Spirit. Ton Ge Ge uses many tea medicines, particularly what he calls "Baume tea medicine" and "Sheep tea medicine." At one time he says he made a hundred bottles of medicine a week. His use of teas stems from his visions in which the Holy Spirit instructs him where in the pastures and fields herbs for curing can be found. Ton Ge Ge treats all types of illnesses in adults and children, including such illnesses as diabetes and circulation problems. He too affirms that prayer is the major element he uses to treat diseases, although he also uses amulets.

COUSAN NOM

Cousan Nom is an herbalist in every sense of the word. He and Noc Sol were the two who provided me with the most information and samples of the medical ethnobotany of the area. It was especially difficult getting Cousan Nom, a distant relative, to respond to my plea for help in furthering my studies. But he finally did. His hesitancy was partly based on a previous bad experience. One of his former patients nearly died, and the family threatened to report him to the health authorities. So Cousan Nom gave up treating others, but he remains an encyclopedia of native medicinal plants.

To be assured that he wasn't quoted he refused being taped, note taking, or photos. He is a nature-loving man who seems to have a bit of sadness in his eyes when he talks about his past experience as a "secret doctor." When I was finally able to get Cousan Nom to talk about secret doctoring, it was during a spur of the moment visit. A very dear friend and close cousin of Cousan Nom took me to his house. He yelled through a truck window that he would join us in the woods to seek out tea medicines (the local term for medicinal plants). He was the expert, and he knew it saying, "you can't find anything without me. You got to know what you're looking for." He had excitedly accepted our invitation; he couldn't resist the opportunity to show us what he knew. He carried with him what he said was his homemade sack, especially made for the collection of plants. He says he and his family strictly rely on herbs and medicines he makes to cure what ails them. The sack was made from an emptied fifty pound feed sack, tied at the two top corners with broken two-inch corn cobs and twine. He also carried a shovel and a knife. When we arrived in what was literally swamps and woods, we began to search out native plants. It was interesting to watch Cousan Nom identify and verify the plants, which initially all looked the same to me. He would say what the native name was, then what it was used for, and how it was prepared in the old days. He then proceeded to instruct me on how to identify them, and at the same time how to be conscious of my environment for any unwelcome creatures, such as moccasins and rattlesnakes. Something basic like a point with a somewhat rounded top on a leaf, in this case snake root, distinguished it from other plants. "It takes time to really learn about plants," he said. After I verified with manuals and documents related to the many plants he gave me samples of, I discovered all were medicinal in some form, and I was in awe of the pharmacopeia knowledge that he and Noc Sol possess.

THE IMPORTANCE OF THIS ORAL HISTORY

These oral histories are the reflections of today's Louisiana African-Americans' attitudes toward illness, the causes of illness, and the importance of religion in its healing. Although much has changed in terms of technology and the advancement of medical science for the African American in this rural population, the folk medicine tradition remains. The main variables affecting health are environmental, cultural, and health services. In an effort to examine the contributing causes of poor health, I will look at statistical data of this community.[1]

In this tri-parish area, there are approximately fifty-nine licensed physicians to every 1,392 persons and 128 nurses to every 628 persons. About 22.8 babies are born per 1,000 in population and 9.9 people die per 1,000 in population in the parish, compared to the 20.5 births and 9.2 deaths on the state average. The fertility rate among Whites in the area is 2.89 and among Non-Whites it is 4.22.

There were approximately 1,301 live births in the tri-parish in 1986, about 18.2 per 1,000 residence. Of those births, 883 were White and 729 were Non-White. Most babies are born in hospitals; however, a small percentage of the population, especially farm persons, rely unofficially on "grannies" midwives. In 1986 four reported births took place outside the hospital, although I know it is not uncommon for a rural Black mother to delay the reporting of a home birth. About 10 percent of Non-White babies born do not reach the age of one. There are three known cases of African-American women aged thirty and below who died giving birth in the early 1980s. Louisiana ranks seventh in the nation in infant mortality. The number of babies who die before reaching their first birthday is 11.8 per 1,000 (Weiss 1990).

A total of 802 people died in the tri-parish in 1986. Two-hundred-ninety-two died of heart disease; 197 of malignant neoplasms; 55 of cerebrovascular disease; and 54 died from accidents. Out of that accident total, twenty-five were traffic-related.

In 1986 there was one case of cholera, seven cases of typhoid fever, fifty-six cases of syphilis, and nine cases of tuberculosis. Cancer appears to be the number-one killer. Lung cancer claims the lives of 17 percent of Black males and 24 percent of White males. Breast cancer attacks 24 percent of the White female population and about 13 percent of Black females. Many Black residents suffer from high blood pressure which results in many illnesses—perhaps the diet consisting of a daily intake of pork, as well as stress-related factors, has something to do with this. A shorter life span and high rates of mortality resulting from illnesses associated with heart disease, cancer, and pneumonia are not uncommon in other African-American populations nationwide (Braithwaite and Taylor 1992).

In rural communities access to a quality medical care is limited, especially for African Americans, Native Americans, and poor people. Prior to 1979 there was only one African-American western-trained doctor in this tri-parish region. He practiced from the early 1920s until his death in 1986. In many cases he was culturally sensitive to his patients' folk beliefs about the causes of illness and misfortune. A colleague once referred to him as a physician that was also a believer and a "non purist of medical science." This doctor confessed that he still came in contact with patients who maintained traditional beliefs about health.

Pinkney says that Blacks historically:

are underrepresented in the health professions. In 1950 some 2.1 percent of all medical doctors in the United States were black, and by 1989 the figure had increased to 3.7 percent. The number of black physicians has historically determined the extent and quality of medical care for the black population because minority health professionals have tended to practice in low-income areas and to serve minorities. (1993, 126)

There are now two African-American general medicine family doctors in the area, including one female. There is also an African-American dentist and a pharmacist.

Secret doctors were patronized more prior to the early 1960s than they are now. The survival of this folk practice is based on the early history of segregation, isolation, and the early harsh medical treatments (which in many cases persist) received from White mainstream medical doctors by Black patients. However, with the recent establishment of medical offices by African-American mainstream medical-trained doctors, more "older" African Americans are employing the services of these Black mainstream doctors. Older persons asserted that their preference for mainstream African-American doctors is because they "trust a black doctor." Furthermore, the African-American doctors are familiar with the cultural traditions of the community. Also, many patients know the family background of the Black doctors, making the bond between Black doctor and Black patient a strong and close one.

Despite technological advancement, folk medicine persists and persons continue to utilize both the folk and the mainstream medical systems. The patient is only interested in what works, and certain factors, such as the cause of illness, socioeconomic status, and access, play a part in determining what medical system will be used (Gould 1957). Therefore, for certain ailments, especially those thought to be new illnesses, the patient goes to the mainstream doctor per the recommendation of the secret doctor. Quite the reverse is true of mainstream doctors in this area. With one or two exceptions, mainstream doctors do not refer their patients to secret doctors for an illness that may be culturally-related. With these doctors, if the patient has a problem related to culture, where historically the secret doctor is known or thought to be the best curer of a specific illness (e.g., childrens' illness, difficulty conceiving), then the secret doctor's care and prescriptions are sought.

One of the problems in rural areas such as this one is access to medical care. Even if certain health care is available, rural African Americans are often reluctant to use these facilities because of cultural biases against mainstream curing methods—surgery, for example. Another type of problem involves the causes and treatment of unnatural illness. In order to understand the causes of unnatural illness, which often are manifested by stress-related disease, one must understand the culture.

Mainstream medical care delivery systems, in most cases, do not adequately meet the health needs of rural African Americans. We can attribute this to cultural differences and ethical discrepancies between the folk medical tradition and mainstream medicine. Furthermore, historical conditions and contemporary realities that have shaped the survival of folk medicine are other factors that must be addressed in a culturally diverse population such as this one.

There are several differences between the medical beliefs and practices of rural African Americans and that of mainstream society. These include: (1) etiology, (2) folk medicine's oral tradition, (3) results of racial discrimination and oppression, and (4) social and geographic isolation.

Medical diagnosis using mainstream medical practices with rural African-American patients tends to be ethnocentric and prejudicial, as it ignores the significance of etiology and cultural values. This cultural relativism phenomenon manifests itself as a struggle between the ideas of what constitutes rational and irrational behavior, relevant and irrelevant cultural values, and effective evaluation.

Significant data (Haskins 1974; Hill 1976; Snow 1977) indicate that a substantial portion of U.S. rural and urban African Americans are consumers of alternative medical care. More precisely they continue to utilize the services of homogeneous folk practitioners—despite growing awareness and access to mainstream medicine. Decisions about where and with whom an ill person seeks medical attention is based to a large degree on cultural factors (Garro 1982). The decision to see a mainstream doctor, or a folk doctor, depends on whether that person shares to some degree cultural similarities.

The data also indicates that utilization of the services of folk practitioners crosses class and literacy boundaries. We find among the patients of secret doctors educated individuals, especially when seeking the services of a mind reader (ethnopsychiatrist).

While women in this area also rely a great deal on folk doctors, they especially rely on women treaters and elderly women to cure and give them advice about problems associated with pregnancy, birthing, and infants and young children. Some of these elderly women were once midwives or have knowledge about granny practices. However, I found it interesting that male doctors appear to be just as popular, if not more so, with female patients who have either reproduction problems or want treatment with reproductive tract complications such as irregular menses.

Thrush, colic, worms, stomach problems, and earaches are common complaints among young children. I found it rather amazing that women of child-bearing age are faithful in utilizing the services of secret doctors for childhood diseases, even though they may not use these secret doctors in any other way. Children are introduced to the power of the supernatural, amulets and herbs, at an early age.

What I found particularly fascinating is that women who do not utilize the services of the secret doctors for themselves will take their babies and young children to them and allow the wearing of amulets. A child's worldview is shaped very early regarding the forces that harm and those that heal. They are taught to respect and have faith in the supernatural. This worldview is reinforced in Christian churches, the major socializing institutions for the society. The church is also the primary reinforcer of the powers of the supernatural—for example, by way of Holy Spirit possession and altar prayer calls. Dramatic healing rituals teach about values and beliefs and offer explanations about who heals and who harms (Mullings 1984). When examining these "social dramas" (Turner 1974), the healing rituals and Sunday church worship, we get a view of historic events that ceremoniously articulate role status, power structure, and African cultural continuity. In this society, then, children learn that God heals, Satan harms, and healing cannot take place unless God is a part of human life and there is fellowship amongst the people.

When we speak of mainstream medicine, for the most part we are referring to the western form of medicine, because it was not until recently that any significant number of Blacks received medical degrees. So when a Black patient says he or she "don't trust no doctor," they usually mean White doctors.

One patient explained that her fifteen year old was having a problem with his genitals (see chapter 2), but finds it difficult to trust white medicine because of historic events which surround the dilemma about Black men's sexual organs and because cultural rituals, such as the rite of passage from boyhood to manhood, are not understood, or they are not viewed in a favorable light by mainstream doctors.

Technological advancement is only recently having an impact on the thinking of the people, and ritual practices for the young prevail. The belief that certain rituals, or rites of passage, must be performed to achieve certain outcomes, such as good health and protection from evil, is prevalent.

There are people, including members of the younger generation, who firmly believe that folk doctors and only folk doctors can cure certain ailments. For example, in one interview I conducted, a thirty-seven year old woman who is the mother of five said, "I took all my children to see 'vieu docteurs de couleur (Old Colored Doctors),' the Colored doctors they know, even the White people come and see them." I have heard many Blacks, on occasion, say they don't go to see White treaters, and White treaters are known to credit much of what they know about folk healing to Black treaters; maybe this is the case because Black secret doctors are noted for their ritual performance.

Today, not everyone in this rural community sees treaters. For certain ailments a treater is consulted, and for more recent diseases, such as cancer, mainstream medicine is consulted. More women today have their babies in hospitals, but some say that women who believe in the old ways are mistreated. Let's say for example a woman (who believes in folk traditions about burying the umbilical cord) may go to a hospital to have her baby but then is denied the "navel string," she then leaves the hospital confused, fearful, and constantly worried, "expecting" something negative to happen to the baby. This kind of anxiety hinders the speedy recovery of the mother, but it also causes guilt feelings, especially if something was to happen to the baby—the mother would blame herself. This anxiety then manifests itself in other forms of disease or illness. This could have been avoided if the mother's folk beliefs were taken into account, especially since this folk practice does not affect the health of the mother, or the child, nor does it endanger others. Permitting the mother to take the umbilical cord with her is an attempt to respect the mother's cultural beliefs.

Ms. Gatts, a White nursing supervisor for one of the Parish public health clinics,[2] stated that babies overall are in better health, but many Black adults still ignore early signs of illness. "Now you see more people with cancer, heart disease and sickle cell, you just didn't see that before," she added. When I asked her if patients who come to the clinic often expressed superstitious beliefs, like wearing the string, she said, "Oh yes, there are still those 'Satan worshippers' who wear the string around the neck for worms and hernia, things like that. But I guess they (mothers) are willing to try anything when a child is ill and he don't respond to medicine." This interview with Ms. Gatts is an example of Black folk beliefs toward health and Whites' attitude toward these Black health beliefs still in existence.

The concept of pain endurance is an interesting one. Although pain is a common indicator that something is physiologically wrong, as Ms. Gatts implied, Blacks tend to ignore these symptoms. This factor often led medical science to conclude that based on differences in skin pigmentations, Blacks had a higher tolerance for pain than Whites as previously mentioned by Langley and Wolff (1968).

Cultural attitudes toward health similar to those previously cited may seem outdated, but the reality is they still exist in this community and other African-American communities in the rural South. Folk beliefs about health are found mostly among persons thirty-five and older—a large percentage of the African-American population.

Foster and Anderson (1978) propose a culture-personality model to study health conditions among indigenous cultural groups where traditional beliefs about illness exist. They feel that because many organic afflictions produce symptoms that are similar to symptoms produced by psychosocial elements, it then becomes necessary to examine mental illness from a psychosocial frame of reference rather than a physiological one.

An example is the case of a sixty-three year old Black female in this community who was diagnosed by a mainstream medical doctor as having diabetes. According to one of my interviewees, this woman never accepted her illness and resented the prescribed treatment, daily insulin shots. Problems of circulation later developed, complicating her health situation. She sought the advice of a mind reader and a treater. The treater performed several spiritual healing rituals and prescribed that she wear the string that he prepared for her. She was not to remove the string, and if she did so the treatment would not work. The woman and her husband visited the mainstream doctor for a medical follow-up. The doctor embarrassed the husband and wife by poking fun at the string and the wife's belief in such backward thinking. The husband was more affected by this doctor's behavior, however. Conflict developed between the husband and the wife and she agreed, for the sake of harmony, to remove the string in order to avoid future embarrassment. The woman's will to get better was destroyed and her condition worsened. She consistently rebelled against mainstream medicine by her unwillingness to adhere to the prescribed treatments and accepted her suffering as one of fate for removing the string. She never regained her health and eventually died.

Psychosomatic illness among African Americans who believe in folk medical practices is not uncommon. Similar examples are cited in studies done by Tinling (1967) and by Lex (1974). These studies indicate that the process of suggestion by a practitioner to a patient who is cognizant of folk etiologies is a powerful antidote to illness or death. According to Jaco (1979), somatic illness and mental health are interrelated. Additionally, he said that health problems related to the mind are not as easily recognizable as those in the area of somatic health; further he found that social change is a major contributor to increased mental pathology.

Social change is indeed a contributing cause of increased stress among this rural African-American population. African-American rural persons' health suffers because of: the socialization process involved as a result of integration; the socioeconomic conditions and experiences of being Black in America (Williams 1974); the feelings of powerlessness and lost values as a result of modernization; the transition from the old to the new way of doing things (such as new ways of earning a living; and having to repress cultural values in order to avoid social stigmas—like wearing amulets, or confining a severely mentally ill family member to a mental institution instead of having the freedom to maintain the mentally ill at home. These kinds of values conflict with the values of the social worker, a mainstream professional, who encourages practices that are more in line with modern treatments. These stressful conditions are manifested into stress-related diseases, such as chronic depression, high blood pressure, cancer, and heart disease.

Studies have shown that social change and technological advancement contributes to increased stress among less advanced communities (Jaco 1979). In cultures that are on the periphery of mainstream culture, stressful living conditions are associated with increased hypertension and/or coronary disease.

Heart disease and high blood pressure are the leading causes of death among African Americans nationally, and it is one of the leading causes of death in this rural community. All these factors—stress, diet, social change, conflicts in values, human variations, etc.—are culturally related and contribute to the process of disease (Underwood 1975).

Another factor which contributes to the maintenance of the secret doctor tradition is the quality of available health care. Because of the lack of trained, sensitive, health care providers, people continue to see secret doctors. "Even today," says Dr. Miles, a member of the National Medical Association and an African American physician practicing in emergency medicine in Louisiana,[3] "only 2% of the total population of doctors in the United States are African American." "Alarming!" she continued, "of this 2% very few are products of rural communities and even fewer understand the folk traditions of rural Blacks because they are usually urban born." "Although some African American doctors may want to comprehend the cultural tradition and are indeed sympathetic, very few actually admit openly to the existence of two medical systems operating in rural areas, and in poor urban areas where there is a high concentration of African Americans. They are thought to view and diagnose causes of illness from a purely scientific point of view, any other approach is going against 'professional ethics,'" she added.

Secret doctoring is usually a major part of socialization for elderly treaters, since they are removed from the responsibility of earning a living. Treaters rely on the practice not as a means of livelihood, but because they are "helping people" and because they are "doing the work of God."

The magical aspects appear to be more popular among the working and lower classes. These classes appear to be less assimilated into mainstream society than an upper-class person. Among upper- and middle-class patients, folk doctors indicate that some believe, but they no longer want to wear amulets or they find a means by which to conceal them.

In Haiti Kiev (1974) observed that therapeutic treatment is often focused on religious beliefs and rituals. Furthermore, relationships between folk doctor and patient in this society, as those in Haiti, are often based on the faith and hope patients have in healing rituals and folk doctors.

This data revealed that prayer, ritual artifacts, and medicinal ethnobotany are key elements which shaped the structure of this tradition. Chapters six, seven, and eight treat these separately.

NOTES

1. Data obtained from the Opelousas-St. Landry Parish Chamber of Commerce.

2. Telephone interview with Ms. Gatts, May 9, 1988, Southwest Louisiana.

3. Telephone interview with Dr. Glenda Miles, April 10, 1988, New Orleans, Louisiana.

4

Madame Neau and Ethnopsychiatry

Mental health maintenance is a major concern among certain African-American populations in rural southwest Louisiana, as well as in other urban and rural African-American communities.

Their folk explanation of mental illness and how to treat it differs from that of mainstream medicine. As a result, many persons from this community seek the advice and care of a mind reader/ethnopsychiatrist, a folk medical practitioner.

In this chapter, I document the life and folk medicine practice of Madame Neau (pseudonym),[1] an African-American ethnopsychiatrist in rural southwest Louisiana. I rely on oral interviews with her, as well as with her son, Doc. The mental health care provider, an ethnopsychiatrist, is commonly referred to in the community as a "Mind Reader."[2] A mind reader/ethnopsychiatrist is the functional equivalent of mainstream medicine's "western psychologist or psychoanalyst,"[3] but the mind reader shares culture and ethnicity with his or her African-American patients (just as the psychoanalyst in most cases shares culture and ethnicity with his/her patients).

As previously mentioned, mainstream medicine defines "health" in terms of pathology—a person free of infection, viruses, or other physical maladies, as determined by clinical tests, is considered "healthy." These diagnoses are primarily based on scientifically-defined results. For communities with folk medicine systems, both mental and physical illness are culturally defined, although Gaines argues that "both folk and professional (medical) systems are equally culturally constructed" (1992, 6).

This folk medical tradition of diagnosis and treatment of mental illness survives among African-Americans, not only in rural southwest Louisiana, but is widespread in other parts of the rural South, as well as throughout the African diaspora (Dow 1965; Kiev 1964; Mullings 1984; Prince 1964; Rogler and Hollingshead 1961). Mainstream medicine is beginning to acknowledge the significance of culture-specific definitions of illness and sickness and are, in some cases, attempting to apply mental health treatment that is culturally based (Campinha-Bacote and Allbright 1992; Capers 1991; Mellette 1979).

Mind readers, usually women, diagnose causes of illness by divining. Divining is customarily done by means of prayer incantations in a trance-like state. This role is similar to diviners in other cultures of the African diaspora and to shamans in Native American culture. Mind readers are insiders (members of the community) who treat their patient's illness according to the local culture's concepts of what constitutes illness and what causes it. Treatments include prayer and lithograph photos of religious saints. In some cases, oils, herbs, and strings are used, but not usually. The lithograph religious photos are the size of playing cards and are carried by the patient for protection, for healing, and to bring good fortune.

Cultural attitudes toward health, similar to those previously cited, may seem "primitive," but the reality is they do exist. Folk beliefs about health in this community are found mostly among persons thirty and older—at least half of the African-American population. Obviously there is a need to address these kinds of cultural attitudes. Going to a mind reader is an ongoing mental health routine for many families in this area.

According to medical anthropologists George Foster and Barbara Gallatin Anderson, an indigenous ethnic group's definitions of mental health should be studied from a culture-personality perspective. This means it is "necessary to examine mental illness from a psycho-social frame of reference rather than a physiological frame" (1978). This chapter is based on just such a perspective, using participant observation[4] conducted with Madame Neau between 1982 and 1984 and interviews conducted with her son (and daughter-in-law) in 1986–87.

HISTORICAL BACKGROUND

Doc, Madame Neau's son, took over her practice after her death. He could not specifically affirm that their practices were African or that healing rituals were historically carried out in a certain manner. He simply said, "this is the way it has always been done." As far as he could remember his mother, and all those before her in his family who were mind readers, practiced this way. This substantiates African-American theologian and cultural historian Albert Raboteau's (1980) claim: theological explanations are not retained in African-American folk religious traditions, but customs are remembered.

The wearing of a mask to conceal or defy true character is a common practice throughout the cultural history of African Americans. Similarities exist in the African-American community's ethnopsychiatric practices, where the practice is conducted in secret. Here, two cosmologies interplay: a Christian perspective and an African one.

Women such as Madame Neau who practice spiritism are also affiliated with the institutional church. Women spiritists, as well as women elders, are regarded as having sound wisdom. They are, in essence, members of the church subpower structure. Most church parishioners (including female and male elders and male pastors) have respect for mind readers and view them as carrying out an aspect of God's work. Outside of the institutional church, in the realm of folk medicine, female and male spiritists are on equal footing.

Mind readers benefit from women's high status within the church and, in turn, create women's high spiritual status. Women mind readers utilize prayer in a very spiritualized "other worldly" way; they rely on their dissociational state, which intensifies the ritual process. This gives the appearance of divine interception. Thus they are often cited as the "most gifted" (intuitive) congregants.

MADAME NEAU'S TECHNIQUE AND ENVIRONMENT

African-American folk medicine is widely misunderstood by mainstream observers. Practitioners express annoyance and dissatisfaction with standard misconceptions that often associate folk healing with eccentric behavior or demonic technique. I am thus revealing an "insider's" point of view, devoid of preconceived biases. In this community, these folk practitioners and their practices are sacred, Christian pursuits.

I was introduced to Madame Neau by a relative of mine. I specifically wanted to observe her treating her patients. On several occasions I became a patient myself. I was especially interested in her appearance, location, counseling procedures, and relationship to patients while treating them. I also wanted to know what she did to heal patients—the questions she asked, her state of mind while treating them, and what "implements" she used (e.g., herbs, oils, powders).

After my initial visits to Madame Neau in 1982–84, I returned to Louisiana in 1986 to record her oral history. I wanted to focus on the folk medicine tradition of which she was a part and her life as a mind reader. When I returned, I was surprised to find a gloomy house. I was unaware that Madame Neau had died the previous summer. Her home had always been alive with the sound of patients' voices spilling from the living room to the street. Madame Neau regularly saw patients from the wee hours of the morning until the sun set in the late afternoon. This was constant—six days a week. "I never practice on Sunday, that's God's day," she once told me.

A neighbor greeted me as I approached the porch steps of Madame Neau's small, wood-frame, shanty-style home early that morning. Her neighbors had always been protective of her. I discovered through conversation with the neighbor that she had died and her son had since replaced her; he would be in later that afternoon. As a result, I obtained much of the information about Madame Neau from her only child and son. He is also a mind reader, who inherited his gift/skill from his mother. This turn of events created an interesting contrast: the participant observation aspect of my research was done with Madame Neau, yet the oral history was provided by her son and daughter-in-law, both "big talkers." Madame Neau, not very talkative, would probably have revealed less. But I did have the opportunity to observe what she did best, counsel.

When I returned, the small living room which doubles as a doctor's waiting room was packed with patients of both sexes and all ages. I was immediately greeted by an attractive, smartly dressed, brown-skinned woman in her thirties. This was unusual—Madame Neau's normal procedure had been for patients to simply come in, take a seat, and wait their turn. I told this woman, the wife of Madame Neau's son, my name and asked if I could see him. I also told her I was doing research, and that I had previously done some work with Madame Neau. She wasn't particularly enthused and grumbled that her husband had this "house full of patients to see" and was occupied with a patient. I assured her I wouldn't take very much of his time. She led me to the kitchen, which was directly behind the living room, and instructed me to wait there.

I waited in the somewhat bare kitchen while she informed "Doc," as she called him, that I wanted to see him. Unexpectedly, Doc came out of the treating room and greeted me. He was about five feet seven inches, with an average build and dark brown complexion. He wore large diamond rings on all eight fingers. I was somewhat surprised by him; his appearance was a bit flashy and totally different from his mother's. She was a rather stout, plainly dressed woman, who always wore an apron, although she perhaps spent very little, if any, time in the kitchen. She always had someone preparing her meals during her working hours. Wearing an apron was part of the general dress code for women of Madame Neau's era. Many women living in this small rural town came from a farming background, and an apron was conveniently worn to serve as a bucket or basket to pick eggs, fruits, and so forth, as they went about their daily chores. The pockets on the apron held Madame Neau's small change, and her bosom held paper money. Certainly, wearing an apron was functional and symbolic of the ordinariness of Madame Neau's character. Madame Neau was also very reserved and meticulous. Doc, on the other hand, was eager and friendly.

I introduced myself and my purpose in the presence of Doc's wife—who was protective of his time and attention. Doc eagerly began to talk about himself, his mother, and the role of a mind reader. He talked for a solid fifteen minutes before his wife, who had returned to the kitchen, interrupted to remind him that he had patients waiting. He agreed to see me later.

When I returned that afternoon, Doc was seeing his last patient. I was directed by his wife to the bedroom Madame Neau had used as her work

space. I sat in the patient's chair, facing Doc, just as I had on previous occasions with Madame Neau. The arrangement of the work space was exactly
as Madame Neau had left it: two chairs facing each other, with a small table
in the center, but not between the patient and the mind reader. The treating
area was in front of a double window, dressed with sheer curtains. This window, which Madame Neau often glanced through, looked out on the street,
the sidewalk, her front porch, and those who came and left. With the exception
of this special corner of the room and various Catholic statues and saints
lithographs, the room was a typical bedroom. Doc's wife sat in on this first
interview and offered her opinions about the mind reading profession.

ORAL HISTORY NARRATIVE[5]

Doc has a doctorate degree in psychology and is an ordained Protestant
minister. After the death of his mother at the age of eighty, Doc relocated to
southwest Louisiana, where he continues to provide counseling services for
his mother's patients. Madame Neau, a renowned mind reader/ethnopsy-
chiatrist, had been "counseling" or "treating" for approximately sixty-three
years. Her patients crossed racial lines and ranged from the poor to well-
known political figures.

Madame Neau was a devout Catholic and a member of the women's aux-
iliary of the Elks. "You must be connected with a church organization to do
this kind of work," Doc says. "Doctors (Western) put you under medication
and make you tell them problems they don't know about. Where we (mind
readers) are gifted through Christ. We don't have to give no medication.
Through Christ we can go back in your past and tell you things you didn't
know about. This is done without looking through a deck of cards, which we
don't handle."[6]

The house where Doc practices is the house in which he grew up. It is in
a working-class, African-American neighborhood located in a rural town with
a population of about twenty thousand. Doc, like most folk practitioners, said
he was called by God to treat. He has been practicing for eighteen years.
Similar to Madame Neau and many folk practitioners in this area, he began
mind reading, also known as treating, at an early age. Doc also refers to himself
in other ways, such as a spiritual psychologist, a healing counselor, and a
doctor of human psychology. "Old people," he said, "that have treated people
in olden days call it spiritual psychology and consider it a gift from God more
than anything else."

Doc is unique—he practices in the same traditional way as his mother,
although he holds a doctorate in psychology. Although college-educated, Doc
makes it quite clear that his knowledge and ability to treat is inherited and a
gift from God. This knowledge preceded college. Madame Neau's harassment
by health officials and other legal entities prompted him to pursue higher
education. He obtained a college degree to avoid similar encounters. Although

he is college-educated, he still treats patients with methods that are familiar to, and culturally accepted by, the community.

Madame Neau saw ten or more patients a day. She treated them mostly with prayer. She prayed silently or mumbled prayers, then went into a trance-like state. This trance-like state was distinctive to Madame Neau and seems to be characteristic of mind readers in this community. "While in this state," says Doc, "the Holy Spirit communicates with the mind reader, and through this communication process he or she is made aware of a patient's past, present and future, their problems and/or illness." While still in this trance-like state, the mind reader is able to diagnose a patient's psychological problem. The treatment process and the extent of the treatment are revealed during this period as well. The average treatment session includes listening to a patient's complaints, problems, fears, and desires; asking questions, advising, and offering solutions. This is followed by a prayer ritual. Depending on the nature of the problem, a typical session may run from twenty to thirty-five minutes. Some sessions have been known to last an hour, but rarely do sessions last less than twenty minutes. A person may be seen one or more times for the same problem.

Doc learned much of what he knows about mind reading by observing his mother in sessions and by listening to Madame Neau's lectures about the power of the mind, the power of faith, and the importance of having a relationship with God. The power of the subconscious mind alone can heal, he explained. "Part of healing," he stressed, "has to do with focusing on an ailment or sore. Some times you don't have to use roots of tea medicine [herbs].[7] The power of the mind is like a person speaking silently to you. You can hear the voice. You go into a stage no ordinary person can understand. They can understand the healing of the physical body, but not the state of mind you're in."

The treatment's success depends on the receptiveness or skepticism of an individual, as well as the complexity of the problem. Examples of the kinds of ailments Madame Neau treated included persons who felt they were having problems or poor health as a result of curse or hoodoo (e.g., a lingering illness, inability to get ahead financially, multiple deaths in the family in a short period of time, constant disharmony in marriages and families). Other patients suffered from natural causes, such as headaches, backaches, stomach problems, circulation problems, bronchitis, tiredness, tumors, and warts. She also provided general counseling to persons who wanted help with decisions and career directions. These included traveling advice, choosing a marriage partner, job choice, and infidelity. If the problem required in-depth treatment, Madame Neau would say various saintly novenas. In addition, she sometimes used healing oils to anoint the person. These substances, usually applied on the wrist and around the forehead, were oils she had mixed and were similar to those found in religious shops. Patients were also often given a small lithograph photo of a saint to carry with them for protection.[8] "For certain problems and situations you have to say certain novenas and prayers," said Doc. "This is one of the most important parts in healing. The novena oil goes along with novenas."

Madame Neau, as is the case with many mind readers, did not advertise her services. Nor did she have a set fee for her labor. However, she accepted monetary contributions, which ranged from fifty cents to twenty dollars. She was called by God to do this work, and she believed a servant of God ought not charge for God's work: it is charity. Often her patient's payment was in kind—a bushel of okra, yams, peas, or the like.

Sometimes mind reading needs facilitation. If the patient is one who is particularly "hard to read" or difficult because of uneasiness, uncertainty, or nervousness, then the patient's hand is used as a guide. Madame Neau's methodology was to position and hold the patient's hand, with the palm facing upward in her own. She used her thumb to press certain points in the patient's open palm. Doc asserted this was not to be confused with palm reading. She used the hand merely as a guide, "just as a student uses a book as a guide." It was a means by which she entered the subconscious of the individual. "The contact with the body and the flow of blood," he said, "is to help determine the problem of an individual who might not otherwise be able to be reached or read."

Doc insists that the gift of treating, although a gift from God, is inherited within families from generation to generation. In each generation there is someone in that family line who possesses the gift of healing, although this gift is sometimes denied or discouraged by certain families. According to Doc, this denial occurs because some are ashamed to identify with the tradition. They do not understand the spiritual and cultural significance of the practice. Doc remarked that "when an individual denies his or her heritage or refuses to accept the gift (folk medical knowledge), their life becomes one of constant turmoil and misfortune, until they accept their heritage and begin to treat (counsel)." This turmoil is viewed as punishment for refusing to carry on the family's folk medicine tradition. This belief is similar to the one related to African-American Baptist ministers. It is believed that if one denies "their" calling to the ministry, then God punishes; only when an individual gives up their worldly ways and becomes a saintly servant of God will their life become more orderly. The same self-sacrificing and pious character is required of mind readers. Within Madame Neau's family line, stemming back to slavery, each generation's matrilineal predecessors were mind readers. Although mind readers generally are women, most families are eager to have the folk medicine tradition survive, and they usually pass on their knowledge to the child with the greatest interest and spiritual intuitiveness—male or female. Girls, however, are often encouraged or persuaded to take an interest. In Madame Neau's case, she had no daughters and very few nieces, none of whom showed an interest in the tradition. Her son, however, expressed an interest in mind reading from an early age. He shared his calling, via visions and dreams, with his mother. He demonstrated his sincerity by spending a great deal of time developing his spirituality and observing his mother.

Mind readers, Doc believes, fill a void left by technological medicine and irreligious lives. "People," he explained,

come to mind readers because they cannot express their problem to no one else. We have sickness in the United States that does not have anything to do with medicine. Sickness come[s] to us because persons are not connected with a religion. We encourage the individual to become affiliated with a church regardless of counseling or our help. There is a difference between Oral Roberts, and people like me, and mind readers. They [Roberts, etc.] only have the gift of spiritual counseling, but they may not have the gift of healing the sick body. Being a [folk] doctor of human psychology, we believe in the Word that can take hoodoo off people.

Hoodoo, according to Doc, does not help people, it only condemns them. "We help those who is convince by this word of hoodoo. We take this word [fear] away from them and we uncross them. And by working against hective work, devils work and witchcraft, we remove them [hoodoo], not put them on you. We take it off." To accomplish this, some old remedies (rituals) that are used are kept secret. "Some [mind readers] tell about it [secret remedies/ rituals]," said Doc, "some don't tell about it, cause they afraid to let too much of it out. They [mind readers] might be misinterpreted into something else that they are not. And people [outsiders] might get a wrong understanding about it." Madame Neau believed that healing was based on faith. The more faith one had, the more help they received from God, and the greater their chances were to be cured of illness and disease. The less faith one had, the less help they received from God and the more difficult it was for a mind reader to help them. This is why she often "prescribed" her patients to attend church, regardless of their denominational affiliation.

CRITIQUE OF DATA

Madame Neau was a highly respected and honored member of the community. I interviewed several persons randomly who were once her patients, or whose family members had been. These individuals, recommended to me through family networks of relatives and friends, had utilized the services of Madame Neau. With them I explored her effectiveness, as well as their attitudes and perceptions of her. Some of these interviewees were leaders of the community and others were regular townspeople. Their opinions are representative of the community.

When I asked Mrs. Marie Santeaux, a former patient, what was it about Madame Neau that impressed her most, she said, "She wasn't a gossiper. She could be trusted. She never discussed your problems with other people." Another patient, Mr. Sam Hosteau, said, "Oh she was good! She could tell you things and most times it was right." Regarding her reputation as a mind reader, Ms. Lotis Guntrie added that because Madame Neau was so effective in what she did, many people were hoping that her son was the reincarnation of his mother. Yet there were doubters. "He doesn't seem to have the understanding about people like his mamma," continued Ms. Guntrie. "He's different . . . he lived away for a while and has that book learning. We'll see how he turns out."

Madame Neau was popular among all classes, sexes, and age groups. Even among educated African Americans, the idea of going to see a Western-trained psychoanalyst still carries with it certain stigmas. The most prevalent stigma is that the person is "coo coo"[9]—the local term for insane. Since no one wants to be thus labeled, they resort to the more culturally acceptable form of psychotherapy, treatment by a mind reader/ethnopsychiatrist.

For patients, protection from natural and unnatural illness and the healing that ensues require certain sacrifices. Thus prayer and affiliation with a local church are often prescribed as remedies for physical and social ills. Prayer-as-treatment is not a new healing concept. In most West African cultures, prayer is used in healing rituals. The belief that one's problems will be solved by "making prayer a habit" and establishing a relationship with the Almighty is common in the African-American religious tradition (Evans-Pritchard 1967; Mitchell 1986). Patients had faith in Madame Neau's "gift" of God, and they credit the folk healer's powerful prayer words with unfailing effect (Oduyoye 1971).

The prayer rituals I witnessed were spiritually intense and effective. Her patients frequently claimed that her prayers had healed them. Another patient, Mrs. Roselle Comeaire stated, "As long as I can remember my family went to see Madam Neau whenever they wanted to know reasons for unexplainable misfortunes and illness." Prayer and spiritual advising were the main services people sought from Madame Neau. Mr. Henri Beggsteau said the healing prayers of Madame Neau cured his teenage daughter of an ear problem. "My daughter was in a car accident," he said. "The accident left her with a serious ear infection which interfered with her hearing," he continued. "I took her to doctor after doctor, but none of them did any good. I finally took her to see Madame Neau. We visited her several times. It was her prayer treatments that finally cured my daughter. She hasn't had problems with that ear since. I am not the only one. I have heard other people say the same thing about her and how good she was."

Privacy during healing rituals is a key characteristic of these southwest Louisiana ethnopsychiatrists—not so very different from mainstream psychiatry. This is confirmed by the location of their work place. Their work place, the bedroom, also assures patients of total confidentiality.

Doc's role as a mind reader is similar to that of a "western psychologist or psychoanalyst." He mainly counsels his patients for their problems. What makes his type of counseling unique are the kinds of disease and illness recognized as counselable by the community. Because the community feels all illness is not associated with medicine, meaning some illnesses are not understood by non-traditional doctors, non-traditional doctors are unable to cure them. Because the patients seem to be particular about whom they can relate their problems to, my guess would be that the mind reader/ethnopsychiatrist must be of a similar cultural background and racial group.

The three kinds of complaints recognized by Doc are: (1) physical illness (e.g., toothache); (2) behavioral or mental illnesses (i.e., those believed to be the result of hoodoo or curse, such as lack of motivation, seeing and hearing things, general bad luck and misfortunes); and (3) complaints that are neither mental nor physical, but simply require general advice (e.g., domestic problems, job choice, etc.). "True" prayer is a petition for material blessings and usually entails asking for protection from evil. It is based on the belief that God is a personal and approachable God (Idowu 1962, 116).

Doc raised the issue about practitioners not being open with their knowledge. This stems from early research done on traditional African-American folk practices by outsiders. The interpretation and labeling (e.g., goofer, conjuring [Puckett 1926]) of the practice has for the most part been negative. In Louisiana in particular, the literature on folk healing tends to relate back to the practices of Marie Leveau and the supposedly wild orgies and sacrificial rites she held on the bayous. These kinds of images automatically provoke eccentric thoughts in the mind of the reader. These terms and tales define the folk customs as bizarre, witchcraft, sorcery, or the like. With these kinds of images, as well as other legal ramifications, one can understand the secret nature of secret doctoring.

QUESTIONS FOR FUTURE STUDY

Religion and magic are closely related to medicine in African and African-American religious traditions. In these traditions people believe that illnesses are the result of natural and unnatural causes. Thus for African Americans in rural Louisiana, syncretic Christian customs, prayer, faith, and the power of the supernatural became the basis for healing rituals.

This chapter raises several issues that have not been fully addressed. More comprehensive study is needed to understand the relationship among the early religious conversion experience of the enslaved African, magic syncretism, and religious syncretism (Bastide 1971), and to determine whether this tradition is predominantly matrilineal in the southern United States, as it has been in certain West African societies. The issue of change and continuity is also an important one. What can we determine about the worldview of the community through its healing customs? And how has the community's worldview changed as a result of outside influences?

Of equal importance are the perceptions of mistrust by these rural Afro-Americans toward western health care systems. It would be meaningful to examine whether that mistrust has contributed in any way to the survival of the ethnopsychiatrist's practice. If so then how worthwhile is it for this community to maintain alternative means to health care as a means of coping with the inadequacies of the Western medical system. That brings us to the role of health policy and its effectiveness or hindrance to a community such as this—hence a need to redefine or implement new policies which address the needs of all its citizens.

NOTES

1. In order to protect the identity of persons in this study, all names are pseudonyms.

2. Mind readers are persons (usually women) whose main function is to divine by means of prayer; in many cases, they may perform healing with prayer. They generally do not use herbs as a part of their remedy. Their role is similar to that of a diviner in other cultures, or a shaman in Native American culture.

3. A psychologist is mainly concerned with the behavior of a person and may have special knowledge about the behavior of the particular group of which the person is a member. A psychoanalyst is more concerned with neurotic behavior as well as non-neurotic aberrant behavior.

4. A participant/observer is one who for the purposes of research goes into a community and spends time with identified interviewees/informants, observing and/or participating in daily cultural practices or in a specific aspect of the culture one is attempting to study. It is different from oral history in the sense that oral history records spoken memories, while the participating observer is on location while his/her informant speaks about the research subject. An informant is an individual(s) who has been identified by the ethnographer/anthropologist as a native authority on that particular aspect of the culture one is researching.

5. This is not a verbatim inclusive narrative. Some things were implied, and some were said but left out in this document.

6. This colloquial speech is common to the area. Doc has not changed his speech habits, even though he has a college education.

7. Tea Medicine is a term used by other treaters in the community to refer to herbs they use in the treatment process.

8. Common saints observed include Virgin Mary (Virgin of Mercy), Saint Miguel (San Miguel Archangel), and Saint Joseph (San Jose). In an interview conducted with Carolina Louisa in Berkeley, California, in December 1987, explanations and comparisons of these saints were made with that of those in the Santeria and Haitian voodoo religious traditions. (The interviewee's father is a Santero [Santeria priest] of Cuban and Puerto Rican ancestry.) She explained that Virgin of Mercy is the equivalent of Oba ta la in Santeria, and although this saint is not directly the patron saint of [physical] health, her use could be associated with the fact that she improves people's general sense of well-being. On the other hand, Saint Joseph and San Miguel Archangel are found in the Congo (Haitian) belief system and are known as Papa Legba, God of Crossroads and Tin-yo in Haiti, respectively.

9. Coo Coo—a person who suffers with a form of mental affliction.

5

African-American Women and Health Care

My approach in Chapter Five is historical and ethnographic. It is concerned with the role of African-American women as health care providers and recipients in light of their own experiences and that of other women in general. This is an important chapter in that literature about rural African-American women in general is practically nonexistent and data on African-American women and health issues is equally scarce.

In this chapter, I first offer a historical overview of women and health issues (drawing from historical and theoretical studies of Blake 1965; Ehrenreich and English 1979; Fee 1977; Lewin & Olesen 1985; Marieskind 1975). I will look at experiences among and between women in general, and African-American women in particular, and how those background experiences reflect differences in sexuality, health attitudes and practices, religious beliefs, etc. This chapter also reveals, through this historical and conceptual discussion about women in health care, that the experiences with the institution of medicine for African-American women differs. Hence, feminist health theories do not provide us with conclusive evidence that explains the experiences of all women. Barbara Christian, in her article "The Race for Theory," explains that western theory is abstract and does not explain conditions of all people. Most theoretical concepts are the assumptions of those "privileged" individuals who get published and in turn whose published manifestos become the voice for all. She goes on to say that people of color have always theorized in their own way—through the oral tradition of stories, riddles, and proverbs (1988).

This language dynamics is eloquently illustrated by the theme of the first National Black Women's Health Project Conference, "I am Sick and Tired of

Being Sick and Tired," taken from the words of Fannie Lou Hamer (Bell-Scott 1985, 2). Christian continues:

dynamic rather than fixed ideas seem more to our liking. How else have we managed to survive with such spiritedness the assault on our bodies, humanity. . . . seldom do feminist theorists take into account the complexity of life—that women are of many races and ethnic backgrounds with different histories and cultures . . . that have different concerns. (1988, 68, 75)

The primary approach in this chapter focuses on the African-American woman's role as provider (folk doctors, midwives, caretakers), and as recipient (patients), in order to determine what constitutes the experience of health, sickness, and health care for them. Angela Davis states, "While our health is undeniably assaulted by natural forces frequently beyond our control, all too often the enemies of our physical and emotional well-being are social and political. That is why we must strive to understand the complex politics of black women's health" (1990, 19).

Historically, African Americans relied on their own traditional forms of medicine, with both men and women serving as health care providers. However, European contact played some part in shaping the meaning of health, illness, and gender among African Americans in religious healing rituals. The Judeo-Christian doctrines also influenced religious values. For example, when the African-American church was organized and in its early years, women were not allowed to serve as preachers. This is still true in the rural Black Baptist tradition. One might argue that status was not diminished, but modified as a result of early Christian assigned roles forbidding women to hold certain leadership roles in the church. After all, African-American women have, since the inception of the Black Baptist church, held leadership positions, often forming their own auxiliaries to advance the causes of women; and, on a broader collective level, they have worked for the social and economic uplifting of the Black community (Brooks 1984).

Unlike the European founders, in the early formation of the Black Baptist churches, African theological concepts acknowledging the high status of women in ritual roles prevailed. The African-American cultural base did not totally abandon traditional beliefs and practices, but modified them by assimilating elements of Judeo-Christian religious practices, initially for the purpose of acceptance by the dominant society and to escape ridicule.

Treating methods utilized Christian prayers, and embodied Christian Gods with African theological concepts. Further, the phenomenon of conversion, divine callings, and possession remain respected as highly desirable attributes for healers. Both women and men are sanctioned into the healing profession based on their experience with these phenomena. Women healers are therefore treated as sacred, powerful, respected, and on equal footing with their male counterparts.

Anita Spring and Judith Hoch-Smith (1978) theorize that "religious ideas are paramount forces in social life, that relationships between the sexes, the nature of female sexuality, and social and cultural roles of women are in large part defined by (that society's religious ideas about women." This concept offers some explanation for the African-American woman's equal footing position as healer. The African-American early Christian perspective was still very much clouded by African theological concepts in which Goddesses were prevalent and powerful entities to attend to. Thus these images, or positions of women, in African theology influenced the sexual function of African-American women. It also determined how women of African descent are viewed in social roles, as well as in participation in rituals.

In the African concept, women healers are viewed as sacred, strong, positive—equally powerful to men as collective community members interested in survival. On the other hand, white women historically, in Judeo-Christian ritual roles as healers, were viewed in a negative light—as unclean, weak, inferior, and malevolent. Because the concepts of Goddesses in African theology are considered powerful, female sexuality was not considered evil where Goddess worship prevailed (the African disaspora). Female ritual images portrayed as one with nature were important to society. Goddesses are associated with water, earth, and views of nature, reflect fertility, growth, food, etc., which in turn mean survival, life, death (ancestor worship).

Nature is an important concept in African society, and a woman's association with nature does not place her in a low status—contrary to suppositions made by some western feminist theorists who considered nature/female a negative female attribute.

In Haitian Vodun for example, "chief (dance) rites extending these beliefs (of nature) are propitiatory and seasonal, ancestral and agricultural" (Dunham 1983). Also, in African-derived dance forms, for example, proper body positions require slightly bent knees and the lowering of the body (torso) as though embracing the earth. "The traditional African dancer," adds Alphonse Ti'erou, "does not attempt to escape gravity or to liberate himself from it but to come to terms with it in order to derive strength from it" (1992). The earth is considered important as it receives the dead; it is associated with food, strength, fertility, nature (trees, hills, sky, sea), and in general considered sacred.

The Judeo-Christian religious traditional concept of women affected the way African-American women are perceived today, not only in their own communities but in the larger society. Early missionary reports and travel accounts reported them as bizarre, evil, wild, domineering, and other negative stereotypical images. These images conveyed African-American women in ritual roles less than human and sought to undermine the validity of the African-American woman's ritual and social role in the religious healing tradition.

Anita Spring and Judith Hoch-Smith (1978) conclude that women outside middle-class western domain retain positions of power and positive roles in ritual domains such as healing rites, midwifery, and possession cults; whereas women in western society, for the most part (not inclusive of all western cultures, e.g., Appalachia), have lost these positions of power and positive images associated with them. Procreative roles, such as a good wife or mother, viewed as positive images, now define western women for the most part.

In the African-American ritual healing tradition, it appears that boys and girls, men and women, may be called or may possess the gift of healing. Women, however, seem to have more intuitive skills than their male counterparts. African-American women are often considered good at divining, and their virtue and utilization of the power of prayer is very pious.

From my observation of women secret doctors in rural Louisiana, they perform the ritual prayer in a state that is between meditative and trance; men secret doctors, though in a contemplative state, usually perform ritual gestures while praying. Women tend to focus mentally and are often said to be more in tune with nature.

In this study women's roles as healers do not vary drastically from that of men healers this leads one to conclude that they are in fact on equal footing. However, in this society mysticism is a standing matriarchal spiritual system. Rural African-American protestant women have exercised Holy Spirit possession for many years as a means of intra-personal communication with God. Holy Spirit possessions and similar states are an acceptable and approved form of spiritual expression by the patriarchs of the Church and the community. This is not an uncommon occurrence, because we find that "the world view of . . . Afro-American societies . . . is such that the altered state of consciousness manifest in the act of spirit possession is highly desirable and ardently sought" (Walker 1980, 29). This form of worshiping is still very much alive in this community. But, as Bourguinon and Pettay (1964) point out, it is difficult to obtain physiological data pertaining to trance states, especially within its sacred context. I experienced avoidance when I asked secret doctors to explain, or describe, the state of mind when actually performing a healing ritual. Nonetheless, I was, in some cases, able to observe this trance state when I was a participant/patient of the healing ritual.

The women who practice traditional healing are members of a Christian church. They are highly respected in the community, and both men and women seek them out for consultation and problem solving. Sabrina Sojourner explains the spiritualism existing among women in African-American religious culture as being similar to practices in other cultures in the African diaspora. She states:

Black theology and folk religion, like traditional African religions, seeks the power or the spirit of God (Divine Energy) in all times and places and things; without that power, one is helpless. . . . By attuning yourself to the Spirit, or its manifestations, you become one with that power. Thus when Black Christians (women) talk about putting themselves in the hands of God, they are generally referring to their need, desire, or ability to tap into a divine source of energy and utilize that energy to push/pull themselves through a situation. This is not much different from the pagan process of channeling energy. (1982, 84)

This explanation may offer some insight to Southwest Louisiana's African-American female practitioners' attitudes toward "other worldliness" and their power with prayer.

In an interview I conducted with Shae and Bae Bae, both women agreed that the character of women healers is symbolic of the rural African-American woman's role as a helper and her connection with the land/nature. What follows is how they describe a female secret doctor's spirituality.

"She could tell you things! She would see things and she was good," Shae said.

"Women are more gifted for seeing things," Bae Bae added. "It goes back to the time when ladies did the helping, and men did the work."

"More men treat. Ladies are more grannies and usually old ladies (are treaters)," continued Shae. "You know its like when people would work in the fields. They believe women use to work the fields. But they only hoed and picked cotton (nurturing tasks). It was the men that was the ones to plow and plant."[1]

This dialogue reflects the communal spirit of gender roles in rural society, but in this case it also indicates the community's view toward the spirituality of women. This "coequal responsibility" conceptually, lacks indepth investigation; however, it is an idea that needs further exploration in order to fully clarify women's role in the dynamics of rural life (Zeidenstein 1979).

In this society, as in others, women are considered the primary cultivators and harvesters of farm crops. They are sensitive, conscientious beings, in contrast to men whose role it is to prepare the land and market the product. Men are believed to be less sensitive by nature, or are not expected to be demonstrative of nurturing qualities. This is an interesting metaphor by Shae and Bae Bae's of land/community use to symbolize human development and sickness and beliefs that women have special spiritual gifts. This African-American cultural tradition teaches its community that women are patient and better listeners. And these are qualities needed in order to be spiritually attuned as a secret doctor, but especially as a mind reader.

Healing is a nurturing profession. In this case the secret doctors are interested in restoring the patients' health. The reap of the harvest is their desire for humankind to have a long and productive life, free of sickness and disease. Women involved in this profession are not interested in economic gain. They are involved because of a genuine love for their fellow human beings. And, because they are not necessarily the primary source of income for the family, they can, usually, devote more time to spiritual development.

Respect for, and association with, nature is found in different genres about

African traditions. In the novels of Toni Morrison, for example, we find this connection with nature and community used in a way to illustrate how this relationship with nature shapes the worldview of African Americans in general, and the perception of women's roles in particular (Christian 1980).

MIDWIVES

As providers of health care, African-American women dominated the field of midwifery in the early history of obstetrics in the United States. This was a specialized skill brought with them from their motherland—Africa. Through-out the history of the plantation-era, Black women functioned in roles as mid-wife "granny." They served as midwives for Black and White women and they were a "prominent personage" (Postell 1951). They were often accompanied by a younger woman who was learning the craft. (Although one secret doctor indicated that men have been known to be midwives as well.) In some cases when another female midwife was not available to assist with a difficult birth, then the attending midwife would call on a man she knew had delivered babies.

Today the midwife's role is changing. In this community, no one openly admits practicing midwifery because it is illegal to practice without a license. But I was told of at least two cases where babies were delivered at home by a traditional midwife. Traditional Black midwives are slowly becoming extinct. Those who are still interested in practicing must meet new state requirements (state board exams, witness the delivery of a certain number of births, etc.). These new regulations make it difficult, if not impossible, for many African-American women to become licensed midwives. There is an active Louisiana Midwives Association, with licensed practicing midwives available to women in rural as well as urban areas (Griffin 1987). Most of these midwives are White however, and Black women view them as they do mainstream doctors.

In this study, the Black midwives' beliefs about health and the birthing process are products of rural communities not unlike those Black midwives in other Black cultures, where populations are usually less then 20,000. Their knowledge about birth and delivery is usually knowledge and experience acquired orally from other women and from being present during a delivery.

In her article, Molly Dougherty (1978) cites many of the roles and functions of southern lay midwives that characterize those in this study. They usually enter the profession as a result of a divine calling just as secret doctors; prayer is usually a part of the treating process; and there are certain taboos that must be adhered to surrounding the birthing process (Boxall 1988; Johnston 1977). The skills and knowledge of midwives are not understood, nor respected, outside of their communities; they are often in conflict and competition with agents who view their positions in the community as a threat, ethically and economically.

Though ideologically similar, nurse/midwives experience less threat, or harassment, from agents outside the community. Nurse/midwives are usually college educated with a nursing degree. One might describe them as nurses who specialize in midwifery and practice in a clinic or hospital, sometimes under the supervision of a physician; this is unlike the lay midwife, who goes to the client's home to practice. In any case, it appears that midwives in general have their own set of problems—lack of support and the low status of their positions.

One approach to confronting these opposing viewpoints is proposed by Mavis Kirkham (1986). She argues for feminist consciousness among midwives who in turn instill self worth in women. Indeed historically midwifery practices have changed over time, making a transition from the domestic to the public sphere (Dye 1980). As a result of segregation and the Black midwife's exclusion from the mainstream medical system, in many cases the Black community received quality health care; because of the Black midwife's healthy attitude about her role, this indirectly had a positive healthy affect on family and the community (Holmes 1985; Schaffer 1991). The credentials necessary to continue practicing was the primary reason for the decline of Black midwifery in various parts of the south.

Historically, cultural studies addressing gender issues in relation to health are ordinarily found in discussions related to white women in particular—their sex roles, family matters, and what has been termed a woman's delicate nature. Women's nature was often characterized as sensitive, intuitive, and emotional; traits that early white patriarchs argued would interfere with the expertise needed for a medical practitioner (Blake 1965). Ironically, these character traits that were held against these early White women healers, placing them in positions of subordination, are the very attributes that are prized for folk doctors in other cultures and should be encouraged in any caregiver.

Recently, however, several scholarly investigations have surfaced challenging the treatment of women's experience and how those experiences are interpreted and presented (Dougherty 1978; Jordan and Kalcik 1985; McClain 1989; Morgan 1989). The literature about African-American women in particular, excluding that on midwifery, and how they perceive their roles as health care providers or recipients is scarce, but some sources do exist (Bair and Cayleff, 1993; Holmes 1985; White 1990).

For the most part early western scholarship stressed the domestic space and the nurturing character of women. In people of color folk medicine traditions, however, women and men folk doctors are on equal footing. Among Mexican Americans, a female curandera (folk doctor) is more highly regarded than her male counterpart (Melville 1980); and in the Native American tradition, the position of a medicine woman is considered one of power and prestige (Jones 1972, Niethammer 1977).

Women's experiences in the realm of medicine are similar, in that women in general have received unfair treatment, particularly as health care recipients. However, women of color's experience with health differs from that of

White women in terms of the high status assigned to women of color healers in non-western cultures. Further, women of color have been victims of medical experimentation (Axelsen 1985; Barroso 1984; Davis 1983; Dillingham 1977; Gonzalez 1982; Hunter 1983–84; Sewell 1980; Shapiro 1985).

Early data indicated that European women too have a history of being traditional healers. However, during the European medieval period, they lost their position as healers to men physicians; women lay healers then became known as "witch healers, practitioners of satanic magic" by the Church and male physicians, who were then advocating scientific expertise and competing for the same clientele.

European lay healing (primarily midwifery and herbology) from its beginning was linked with nurturing—qualities commonly identified with the character of women. The early church condoned scientific and condemned traditionalist expertise arguing that women were evil and inferior. Witch hunts were enforced to eliminate women lay healers. An important aspect of scientific health care providers' training was based on philosophy and early folk Christian concepts and practices which included magic, while the lay healers' training was based on the oral tradition passed from generation to generation (Ehrenreich and English 1979).

With the emigration to America came lay and scientific practitioners; however, violence was no longer used to outlaw lay practices. Rather capitalism became the major focus of health and health care delivery. Medical care now had to be purchased—payment in exchange for services, now mostly provided for by men. Women's experience as providers was now limited to the immediate family and community.

According to Lewin and Olesen (1985), the concept of women's health entails being concerned about the well-being of women and assuring that women are informed about health issues so that they can have control over their health status and bodies and be able to make choices about them. The more recent women's health movement emerged in the early 1970's advocating that basic idea. It was a movement primarily concerned with a need for women to liberate themselves from social oppression and to fully understand the health care process. Specifically, it addressed alternatives to medical care, advocated preventive health concepts, self-awareness, knowledge of body, and the demystification of medicine.

Its goal was to seek improved health care for women and end sexism in the health care system. It was a social vehicle for women from various socioeconomic backgrounds to come together collectively to discuss unsatisfying experiences with health care. Assumptions made by the movement included that the social oppression of women was based on biological differences between men and women, and on women's ability to reproduce. Those differences, which are the social foundation of female subordination and male domination in society in general, are the same factors that control the male doctor/female patient interaction within the context of medicine (Marieskind 1975).

Although the National Women's Health Network was organized with the intent of representing the needs of all women, many women, especially African-American women argued that the goal of the women's health movement ignored, or excluded, the concerns and special needs of African-American women. Further, that efforts to change socialization of female/male roles in society, or that of health care providers, was insufficient if there was an absence of cultural sensitivity on the part of those who sought sisterhood. Thus emerged the National Black Women's Health Project.[2]

The issue of exclusion[3] and the need for self-help were the motivating reasons for the formation of the National Black Women's Health Project (NBWHP), the fastest-growing women's organization in America. Located in Atlanta, Georgia, the NBWHP was formed out of a need to address specific health care issues of African-American women. Conceived by Bylly Avery, who had begun work with the National Women's Health Network, the NBWHP was organized in 1974. Its beginnings focused on abortion and gynecological care, and later grew to include prenatal and alternative birthing.

The NBWHP stressed the holistic approach to health care. It addressed specific issues, which in some way have a direct or indirect bearing on the health of Black women—economics, cultural differences, prenatal care, infant mortality, environments of trust, language use, support network, violence and sexism, were all issues of priority. These were very basic concerns centered around survival as a result of one's race, gender, economic status, and as victims of oppression. Avery also felt that the conspiracy of silence was the result of the power structure's attempt to silence the voices of Black women by exclusion in the literature, and to create silence within the Black community. "It's about black women making their voices heard. Health is mental, physical, and social, it is about talking it out, talking about it and doing something about it" (Avery 1990). Until the founding of NBWHP, no organization specifically addressed health concerns of Black women. Nor did anyone lobby for their special concerns.

BLACK WOMEN AS RECIPIENTS

Various factors affect women as recipients of health care. Some of the early attitudes toward White women from White medical practitioners surely have had a direct, if not indirect, effect on Black women who are viewed in much the same way—from a sexist perspective. These factors determine how a woman interacts with a doctor and how a doctor interacts with her, the kind of medical care (diagnosis and prescribed treatment) she receives, the quality of the care received; further, how a woman views her body, or how others view her body, will determine how responsible she is in seeking care (Ehrenreich and English 1979; Martin 1985).

For African-American women the problem of quality health care is magnified. Not only are the factors of image, sexism, classism, and all of the concerns we have mentioned for women in general a reality, but they are compounded by racism and cultural differences making quality care, or whether a Black woman receives care at all, even more complex.

Factors such as race, gender, and socioeconomic conditions put African-American women at greater risk of poor health. According to Gordon-Bradshaw (1987), such factors place these women at a very high risk of being victims of subservient and inadequate health care. Those living in poverty are more concerned with basic survival needs, and preventive health care measures, such as pap smears, breast exams, etc., are not a priority.

On the other hand, there are cultural factors (diet, trust, etc.) that are equal determinants for quality care. In an article appearing in *Essence* magazine, an African-American female patient explained her encounter with a mainstream medical institution, an experience that is characteristic of many African-American women. "These doctors are racist and sexist. . . . If you're poor, minority and on Medicaid you don't get the same kind of treatment. We are expendable. I waited seven hours in the emergency room. They would never do that with a white woman." The author (Freeman 1991) goes on to say that although serious illness is more common among blacks they "visit physicians less often, are hospitalized less frequently and are more dissatisfied with health care than white Americans of similar socioeconomic status."

These multiple hazards are even worse for rural African-American women; their poor health care is often a result of their rural and minority status. Rural women in general have special concerns and problems that are often related to restrictive finances, isolation, lack of physical access and availability of health care, lack of insurance, etc. (Richardson 1987). One might conclude then, that to be a rural, poor, African-American woman is suicide or at least self-destructive. Data on poor rural women are limited, and almost nonexistent for rural African-American women and other rural women of color.

Certain health conditions are more prevalent among rural women—arthritis, back disorders, bursitis, hearing and visual impairments, ulcers and hernias—conditions that are related to the requirements of maintenance of rural environments and farming. Rural women are also less likely to have funds or other means to pay for medical care, as insurance is a luxury for many rural families. Medicaid and medicare, although designed to meet the needs of the poor, often exclude self-employed farm women or those who for other reasons do not meet the criteria to qualify for medicaid. Yet most are financially unable to afford monthly insurance premiums.

In one interview I was told of a situation where a woman and her husband had inherited a small farm from their parents, and now farming was their livelihood. However, the woman became chronically ill. After exhausting the couple's cash flow augmenting their limited health insurance coverage, the woman was forced to seek other means of medical care. She discovered that the home and property they owned disqualified them from receiving social security benefits, even though their income was below 12,000 dollars. To further complicate matters, she was told that she did not qualify for disability because of the combination of her age and lack of contributions into the social security system (as a self-employed farmer). As a result of her inability to obtain outside social services help, she only sought medical care when absolutely necessary—when she was near death. This is not an uncommon occurrence for rural families, and certainly it is magnified among African-American families who live in constant fear of losing their homestead.

Leith Mullings argues that the Western concept of medical knowledge is often based on the cultural view of women's place in society, hence diagnosis and treatment reflect this sentiment (1987). That is, a woman's complaints are unimportant if there are no obvious signs of illness. Diagnosis of female disorders were often associated with a woman's nature or sexuality. For African-American women, their place in society as women is also determined by the position of their race in society—that is as a subordinate minority group; thus she and her ailment is treated subordinately.

The African-American woman brings her own special baggage of stigmas attached to being a Black woman, which further contributes to attitudes toward the Black woman as a patient. Historically, the perceptions are a carryover from the time of slavery toward the sexuality of African-American women. Early accounts stigmatized Black women as being promiscuous and breeders (Gilkes 1983; Gutman 1979; Ladner 1976). The early stereotypes play an important part in shaping the present day perceptions of Black women by mainstream medical professionals. Such stigmas influence health care decisions about Black female patients, limits health care choices for Black women, makes trust of mainstream medical practitioners questionable, etc. These kinds of attitudes toward Black women makes the provision of health care for them—especially low income, rural women—unfair and inadequate. Medical decisions have been based on these misconceptions, resulting in patterns of treatment such as unwarranted sterilization procedures as a means of birth control.

Several studies have been done to determine if physicians view and treat women and men patients differently. One study concluded that the manner in which a woman expresses a problem to a physician will determine whether she receives treatment or not, or whether the physician views the problem as an overexaggeration. Conclusions made by this first study suggest that women patients demand more of a physician's time than male patients, and that women's complaints were more likely influenced by emotion, thus being characterized as psychosomatic (Bernstein and Kane 1981). Another study found that women were more likely to receive more "treatment" than men—finding that women overall are more likely to receive more laboratory tests, drug prescriptions, etc., assumably due to physicians' sex bias (Verbrugge and Steiner 1981).

Factors such as race, class, and sexism influence health care providers' diagnoses; as a result the longevity of Black women is affected because the women refrain from seeking medical attention unless in a crisis. More research is needed to fully understand the impact these variables have on the well-being of women who are rural, poor, and persons of color. More research is also needed to adequately assess what approaches are needed to address the complex health needs of this population (Bassett 1986; Bushy 1990; Lawhorne 1990; Satariano 1986; Zambrana 1987).

There are special risk factors that are indigenous to African-American women. Although fewer Black women have breast cancer, more Black women than White women die from breast cancer or cancer of the uterus/cervix. Research studies cite as the reason, Black women's lesser likelihood to seek preventive measures such as mammography and pap smears. Hypertension, which leads to diseases such as heart failure, strokes and kidney disorders, is another risk factor that is more prevalent among Black women. Obesity and malnutrition are also high among Black women—risk factors that lead to increased danger of mental disorders, diabetes, colon cancer, and depression as a result of distorted body images (Cope and Hall 1985). And, the lifestyle of Black women is generally high risk. Dangers of smoking, alcohol and drug abuse, violence in the home and community, and the impact of stress, all contribute to the alarming high-risk health factors found among Black women. All of these determinants have a direct correlation to the quality of life for the Black woman, the Black family, and the Black community (Malveaux and Simms 1989).

Hilda Richardson (1987) maintains that regardless of the place of residence, the lower the income the more likely women are to experience poor quality health; but rural women are especially affected by elements such as a lack of transportation, isolation from health care resources, shortages of health care personnel, emergency services and hospital beds, that contribute to the burden of access to quality health care.

Some feminist scholars, such as Fee (1977), theorize that one reason for the condition of women's health is women's position of social subordination in society and inequality in employment and education. Although women are a majority in health professions, they, as well as people of color, are a minority in decision making and administrative roles in health care.

As recipients, African-American women have historically had little to say about the kind of medical treatment they received, and they have often been victims of involuntary sterilization—an occurrence that has also been a part of Puerto Rican (Lopez 1987) and Native American women's history (Clarke 1984). According to reproductive rights activist Adele Clarke, subtle forms of sterilization are on the rise. She states:

Sterilization abuse, the coerced or unconsenting sterilization of women and men occur in both blatant and subtle forms. Blatant abuse includes forced sterilization against a person's will, sterilization without telling the person they will be sterilized, and in the United States sterilization without the patient's informed consent to the procedure. Subtle sterilization abuses include situations in which a woman or man legally consents

to sterilization, but the *social conditions* in which they do so are abusive—the conditions of their lives constrain their capacity to exercise genuine reproductive choice and
autonomy. (1984, 188–89)

Angela Davis (1983) concludes that the issue of involuntary sterilization
didn't come to the fore until 1973, with the incident of the Relf sisters in
Alabama. In this case two African-American girls, ages twelve and fifteen, were
blatantly sterilized. African-American women have been characterized as
"baby machines," a stigma that is a contributing factor to the erroneous ra-
tionalization of blatant or subtle sterilization. Davis cites a 1939 statement to
address birth control among African-Americans from the Birth Control Fed-
eration of America, "(t)he mass of Negroes, particularly in the South, still
breed carelessly and disastrously, with the result that the increase among
Negroes, even more than among whites, is from that portion of the population
least fit, and least able to rear children properly" (1983, 214).

These same perceptions prevail today. As recently as 1991, a professional,
White, female student commented to me that she worked with Black teenage
girls, and in her work she encountered many Black teen pregnancies. Further,
for the most part, the girls did not believe in birth control—a fact she couldn't
understand because most of these girls were not equipped to become mothers.
She added that financially they couldn't afford to have a baby, because the
fathers of the babies were absent. These pregnancies then result in an enormous burden on the welfare system.

Her reasoning was not uncommon, nor unusually irrational, nor was her
perspective ordinarily insensitive nor different from the perceptions and remarks made on a mass scale toward low income parenting. What baffled me
most was her follow-up comment about the solution to the problem. This
White female student stated that her most recent advisee, a fifteen-year old
African-American girl, an AFDC mother who now had one child and was
pregnant with a second, was not sure whether to have this second child. Her
response to this example of a perplexing situation was "she is a perfect candidate for (unknowing) sterilization." She proceeded to explain that she recommended abortion to the fifteen-year old girl, but was adamant that the
fifteen-year old needed to be sterilized. Being incapable of reproducing would,
in the mind of the White student, resolve a fifteen-year old child's problems
about sexuality and end the cycle of poverty and welfare dependency among
Black single female-headed households.

Poverty is a primary factor interfering with African-American women receiving proper care. In this study many of the women consistently complained
that one of the many reasons they seek the care of a secret doctor is because
of the high cost of health care and because of mistrust of white mainstream
practitioners. Wilkerson and Gresham (1989) argue that the phrase feminiza-
tion of poverty, a phrase used to define the high concentration of single
women-headed households living in poverty, is the racialization of poverty.

Racism, they conclude, a key barrier to employment opportunities for African Americans, is the cause of poverty. They further contend that the welfare system blames these women for having babies outside of marriage, but fail to take into account that the fathers' noncontribution to the family is largely based on his (un)employment status and the historical exclusion of Black males (and women) from opportunities for economic success.

According to Wattleton (1990) teen pregnancy in the United States is higher than any other westernized country; but data indicate that the determinant of teen pregnancy overall, is class-related, rather than race-related. In the African-American community, teen pregnancy is just as much as a dilemma as social exclusion and impoverished conditions. Sterilization, "sexuality education and family planning services cannot solve the teen pregnancy problem. . . . society must provide all our young people with a decent education, tangible job opportunities, successful role models and real hope for the future" (1990, 111).

Sterilization is not a choice, and many women (especially teenage girls) do not fully understand the permanency of the procedure; yet, many medical care institutions and workers continue to manipulate a large percentage of low-income girls and women into believing that it is indeed a solution as a means to control the sexuality of poor, women of color.

NOTES

1. This statement does not necessarily mean women only hoed crops and picked cotton; quite the contrary, rural African-American women shared in all of the farming chores, including harvesting sweet potatoes, corn and other crops, as well as performing other duties. Nor does this statement imply that African-American men only plowed and planted. This is a metaphor of sorts to illustrate not only the communal spirit of gender roles, but that African-American homestead women indeed had clearly defined functions and roles that perhaps is not very clear to outsiders. Further, these roles were viewed as important and high status.

2. An extensive interview conducted with Loretta Ross, National Program Director of the National Black Women's Health Project, gave me some background on the development and mission of the NBWHP.

3. Elizabeth V. Spelman, author of *Inessential Women: Problems of Exclusion in Feminist Thought* (Boston: Beacon Press, 1988), challenges White feminist theorists to examine their record in terms of their own treatment of women, especially women of color, in which they will find that the cycle of exclusion is being repeated by White middle-class women who treat other women as inessential.

6

Religion, Prayer Narratives, and Healing

The African-American religious tradition in this rural community is characterized by Baptists and Catholics whose theological beliefs are based on orthodox religious doctrines and nonorthodox religious healing customs that are simultaneously practiced. African-American religion is a structure based on the old, traditional West and Central African theology and customs, and the new (Christianity) (Baer and Singer 1992; Barrett 1974; Pitts 1993; Raboteau 1980; Simpson 1978; Sutton 1983).

The Christian perspective "provided a language for the meaning of religion, but not all the religious meanings of the Black communities were encompassed by the Christian forms of religion" (Long 1986, 7). Some aspects of folk medicine, for example, could not be communicated via Christian forms. Where this was the case, the African perspective came into play. Religion for African Americans, particularly among protestant fundamentalists, functions to "compensate for the daily subservient and emotional restraints imposed upon them" (Gray 1979, 19). The protestant denominations offered the African an acceptable means by which to release emotional stress. It is not surprising that often part of the remedy the secret doctors prescribe for their patients is fellowship with others. Also Holy Spirit possession is still encouraged and viewed as therapeutic. In African-American culture, the church, Bible, and clergy are viewed as a composite healing institution—one that functions to reinforce self-worth (Fisher 1988; Smith 1976).

Is this ethnomedicine tradition magic based, or is it religious based? According to the Western definition of magic, some early religious forms have their origin in magic, and world religions evolved from magic. Faith is magic;

people put their faith in God's hand. Prayer, too, can be characterized as a magical formula. When we seek to manipulate or control a situation, we sometimes recite this formula—we pray.

Among some earlier mainstream scholars (Frazer 1922; Tylor 1920), medicine, magic, and religion were thought of as inseparable. It is common practice among most cultural scientists today to view medical beliefs within the cultural context of religious attitudes and magical practices.

In this society, a child's world view is shaped very early to respect the supernatural and benevolent and malevolent spirits. Children are taught the importance of striving to keep a balance between self and others because "the devil (Satan) is always trying to take over." Since the devil is such a powerful malevolent force, the aim is to always remain in good standing with God and the church—benevolent forces.

Any breach of taboo, a long absence from church for example, creates a disharmony and is a fall from the grace (protection) of God and community. Without protection a person becomes vulnerable to the forces of Satan (misfortune, bad luck, death, and sickness). The role of family and community, and the need to promote harmony between individual and society (social control), as a means of healing is important. Thus, beliefs about illness cannot be comprehended outside the cultural context of the community.

This religious fervor of African Americans is quite different from White Christianity. White Christianity does not consist of the same kind of community bond and need for salvation. In any case, mainstream medicine is a capitalistic venture. The rural Louisiana African-American folk medical system, on the other hand, functions as a healing institution, as well as a means to control social behavior and support cultural norms.

Magic, religion, and medicine have often been referred to in the same context and in some ways their domains overlap. Rivers offers a provocative explanation of this concept based on acculturation. He says:

When we find a mode of treating disease closely related to a magical or religious practice, it becomes possible that the relation does not represent a stage in a process whereby medicine is gradually being differentiated from magic or religion, but the process may be rather one of assimilation.... we have a highly complex process of interaction between peoples and their cultures, producing blended products ... blends of medicine with magic and religion. (1924, 60)

This theoretical assumption can be applied to the healing phenomenon in this rural farm area of southwest Louisiana and in other studies on African Americans done by Hill (1973, 1976), Hurston (1983), and Snow (1977a, 1986), where magical aspects of prayer and scriptures are essential to the efficacy of the healing ritual.

Two elements are key in illustrating the cultural continuity and the relationship between folk medicine and other religious aspects in the community—the belief in the power of the supernatural and prayer.

NATURE AND FUNCTION OF PRAYER

Prayer has healing affects. According to Carter (1976, 80–81), "for Black people healing is definitely achieved through prayer. . . . Black people do not seem to draw any firm line between mind and spirit, soul and body. They believe that healing reaches the total person. They carry with them the belief that . . . God's man, can 'get a prayer through' where others will fail." God's wo(man) in this case is the secret doctor, who is called, just as the minister, by God, to doctor. The patient believes that secret doctors are "gifted" with special powers to interact with the Supreme Being. Patients believe that secret doctors possess special powers, and that their prayers bring about results where the lay persons' prayers have failed.

All prayers in this study are religious types and begin with invocation. There are three kinds of prayers employed in healing endeavors. They are (1) prayer proverbs, (2) secret prayers, and (3) call and response prayers. The prayer proverbs and the secret prayers are those found in the healing rituals of secret doctors. The call and response prayers are found in prayer meetings. These prayer meetings, in most cases, are for the purposes of healing, and they fall under the umbrella of the institutional church. All prayers are individual, hence variations may occur.

Research conducted on the prayer experience is limited. However, in a study conducted by Poloma (1991), various prayer activities were surveyed and categorized into four types: (1) ritual prayer—is a prayer that is read from a prepared script or reciting a memorized prayer; (2) conversational prayer—a prayer that involves having a dialogue with God; (3) petitionary prayer—a prayer that is said in a state of crisis and is a direct request to God asking for help; and (4) meditative prayer—involving thinking, feeling, and listening to the presence of God. Themes and functions of prayer do seem to have similarities cross-culturally, although differences exist. I was especially interested in Metcalf's (1989) examination of the place and meaning of prayer in religious ritual.

There are other prayer contexts directly or indirectly related to healing (e.g., the altar call prayer), however my study is limited to the three formerly mentioned types used in healing. Prayer functions as an expression of the religious faith of the secret doctors and the patients who come to see them. The secret doctors say they are believers and their patients must also have faith in the prayers or they won't be healed.

SECRET PRAYERS

The secret prayers are in most cases passed on in Creole French. They are the Our Father or a formal Catholic prayer, and they are usually said silently or mumbled. Secret prayers are also said when the patient is not present, such as in the continuation of a healing ritual (Beedeau prays at his altar for patients). They are prayers that are common among the French-speaking Catholic and Baptist communities. What remains secret, and is not common knowledge, is what prayer is said when and for what illness. Obtaining significant data about these prayer texts was impossible.

Very little is known about these prayers—Why certain prayers are selected for certain illnesses? Why are they said a certain number of times? Why is it necessary to recite these prayers in Creole French? Why are they considered secret—just how many of these secret prayers exist is also not known. In the Yoruba tradition, it is also common for certain aspects of ritual ceremonies to remain secret, such as "applied literary art forms" (prayers, folktales, myths) (Bascom 1953, 130).

One may speculate on several reasons why the prayers are kept secret. One reason is the concept of power. If only a few people have knowledge about a remedy, then it makes them the authority and a controlling force. In Liberia, for example, certain remedies are known by all people of the Poro and Sande societies, and then the prayers thought to be most valuable are only known by healing specialists (Harley 1970).

Another contributing factor to prayer secrecy could be that certain prayer petitions needed to be kept secret from the European powers in control at the time. A prayer petition for a person who was bitten by a snake while trying to escape is an instance needing secrecy. In addition to praying for the wound to heal, the secret doctor would ask God to help the escapee with a speedy recovery so that he or she is more successful with the next escape attempt.

In any case, probably the most important reason for secrecy in prayer is associated with power and control. Not everybody can be a folk doctor, nor do they meet all the prerequisites to deserve the title; so naturally wisdom associated with the profession is reserved for a select few. As one interviewee said, they must pass the test of "time and spirituality," otherwise they may misuse the knowledge.

PRAYER PROVERBS/SAYINGS

The prayer proverbs are short improvised petitions. For these prayers, the content applies to an individual situation and illness. There are no specific nor predetermined words. The manner in which words for these prayers are said do appear to have some pattern however. Information about what words these prayer proverbs contain and how they are said was obtained with a certain amount of ease.

The prayer proverbs were silent, or mumbled, and they were not memorized nor formulized. They are similar to what Evans-Pritchard (1967) calls a saying. It is comparable to the kinds of prayer sayings/proverbs that the Mano ethnic group of Liberia say when anointing curative amulets they give to their patients.

Details of the prayer sayings differ and are based on each particular client's situation. A typical example of a prayer saying for a person with ulcers follows (according to a Louisiana secret doctor): "Dear God, help (person) be rid of this awful disease, bring health back to (person) stomach, etc." Similarly the Mano folk doctor prayer said for protection of a blacksmith opening a new shop states: "Let everyone who comes to work here have good luck. Let the smith of this shop prosper and get plenty of work. Let him live long. Let his Children be healthy," (Harley 1970, 173).

Other examples of prayer sayings include two prayers collected from a local folk doctor in a study done by a student at the University of Southwestern Louisiana.[1] There appear to be specific prayers for specific illnesses but they too are characteristic of saying prayers. For sunstroke, or any illness related to burns or burning sensation, the prayer is repeated nine times: "The sun, in the name of the Father, Son and Holy Ghost, I command you to come out of this person as quickly as you went in." The other prayer is a prayer that is said for bleeding and it is said seven times: "Blood, blood, I command you, in the name of the Father, Son, and Holy Ghost, to stop bleeding and I put you in a pumpkin and cross the water."

The African-American prayer tradition of southwest Louisiana is not totally unlike those of people and folk doctors in West Africa. "Above all, prayer is essentially an asymmetrical relationship with a supernatural power perceived in experience. . . . healing is an activity second only to that of giving life. Petition for healing is the most common subject of prayer in the African tradition," says Aylward Shorter (1975, 61). Shorter cites a prayer by a medicine man from Kenya. It is similar to the previously mentioned prayer proverbs. "Nyaga help his man that he may be well, that he may recover tomorrow, and may you want to help this man to be well; and, as overcoming you overcame, overcome all these troubles, and have mercy on me, because we do not know how to pray to Murungu, [Different] from what we say now."

CALL AND RESPONSE PRAYERS

The call and response prayer is typical of most prayers in prayer meetings of African-American churches. Essentially what takes place is group praying. One person prays, from a group perspective, but with a focus on individual petitions. The other members of a prayer meeting respond and support those petitions. Then another person prays with the same prayer structure but with a different content. This cycle is repeated until all have prayed who wish to do so or until the designated number of prayers have been said. The call and response prayer is examined briefly because prayer meetings are no longer recognized as an official healing ritual. In addition to requests for healing, people now attend prayer meetings to ask for divine Providence, give thanks, etc.

Two edited versions of selected prayers from a prayer meeting are included in the notes.[2] These are call and response prayers and are good examples of prayers focusing on health and healing of the physical and spiritual body, as well as of the mind. The meetings for these particular prayers were held in a local Baptist church. Some prayer meetings are still held in homes; if a member is ill, homebound, or bedridden, then the "prayer band" goes to the sick. One prayer is by a sixty-five year old woman and the other is by a forty year old man. The content and style are the same. Prayer closing is usually mumbled statements of praise and private petitions.

The formalities of the prayer meeting begin with the usual opening: a praise song, then a devotional response by the chair of the prayer meeting, followed by the usual announcement indicating the number of prayers to be prayed and assigning individual persons to pray. Another method of conducting prayer service is to open the floor to anyone who wants to pray. In this case a prayer meeting can last the usual one to two hours, or the unusual three to four hours, depending on the number of people present and the number desiring to pray. But in all cases, anyone can pray if he or she so desires, simply by calling out, "prayer continue."

There are no distinctions made between women and men. Any woman present, or any man present, is allowed to pray. I did notice, however, that the women tended to sit together with women and the men sat with men. This is not entirely uncommon because it is the normal seating arrangement on Sundays during church services, particularly among older members.

The content of the prayer and the performance of the prayer text does not differ greatly between men and women. Early data indicates that women have always participated freely in the African-American prayer tradition (Donald 1952). This study confirms that even in today's contemporary setting, Black women are a very viable part of the African-American prayer tradition. Prayer ministry in the church is often led by women leaders of the church. Such persons as church mothers (also referred to as deaconesses or steward sisters) "minister to persons in the general areas of healing." These women owe their talent for this skill in praying and psychic reading to the "inherited role of the African priestess" (Carter 1976, 78–79).

All who pray are usually in a kneeling position. One difference between women and men who pray is that the women are not as vocal, or physical as the men, meaning the men's voices are louder and they tend to move around more while on their knees. This is not the norm for women, who are rather reserved with their bodies. Perhaps they are conscious of their role as women and the image they portray. I might add that some of these same people who attend prayer meetings see secret doctors.

PRAYER THEMES AND STYLE

The most common themes found in these healing prayers are characteristic of those categories defined by Shorter (1975). One theme is for divine governance. This theme glorifies the power of God, and it is present in all prayers of healing. Another theme is for health and healing. And a third theme is the request for divine protection. These too occur in all healing rituals.

Prayers are oral and long, or silent and short. In most cases, they are accompanied by ritual gestures. For example, in the case of a healing ritual for a woman suffering with a series of miscarriages, the secret doctor, in addition to prayer, circled her abdomen several times with his hands but never touched her. The healing prayers start with an invocation, a statement about the problem, followed by a request for help in solving the problem, and conclude with praise to the Almighty as having all powers.

There are no set times for secret doctors to say these healing prayers. This may vary from secret doctor to secret doctor. One secret doctor says that in addition to praying while the patient is present, he also prays at his altar in the mornings. This method is perhaps an individual technique rather than a standard traditional practice for secret doctors. On the other hand, prayer meetings are scheduled, and they are usually held at night. The mornings were cited as the time for prayer meetings held when making requests for rain. The call and response prayers are very similar to the prayer oratory of the Georgia Sea Islands' prayer meetings, where the invocation begins with the Lord's Prayer (Jones-Jackson 1987).

Although the call and response prayers are spontaneous, the basic style is consistent with tradition. In healing rituals, secret prayers are memorized prayers. Prayers cited as secret prayers were the Our Father, the Hail Mary, Act of Contrition, and Confess Almighty God. In order to learn the secret prayers, a person must have good a memory and speak Creole French.

HISTORICAL FACTORS OF PRAYER

The Catholic prayers said in Creole French seem to be a part of a historical tradition. These are prayers passed from generation to generation. Also inherited is the style and structure of the ritual prayer—the manner in which they are said and performed. These prayers and the "old time religious prayers" often heard in prayer meetings are prayers that are very effective in exciting emotional response (Pipes 1951).

Because some of these prayers are passed on in the original language, Creole French, and some are Catholic, perhaps they originated around the time of the French rule and the dominance of Catholicism in Louisiana. It is not at all uncommon to find Baptist people practicing Catholicism, that is, refraining from eating meat on Fridays, making the sign of the cross, etc. Catholic influences also dominate Baptist traditions in other communities in Louisiana (Jenkins 1976).

Prayers employed by secret doctors in rural southwest Louisiana are to protect as well as cure. Protection requires certain sacrifices associated with treatments prescribed by the treaters, such as periods of daily intense prayer and attending church more often (fellowship). Prayer is not a new phenomenon, and it appears that there is a renewal in attitude toward prayer and the power of prayer and faith as more contemporary persons seek spiritual guidance through it (Barnhart 1988; Droege 1991; Ojoade 1986; Stuart 1989; Winston 1990).

Attending prayer meetings are an important addition to the healing tradition. These prayers are said for thanksgiving as well as for healing purposes; the prayers are for individual healing of the body and mind, as well as for communal healing. The petitioners ask for personal health, family health, and good fortune. In addition the prayers ask for improved social relationships in the community, a stronger church family, and blessings for everybody.

I asked one minister in the Community, Rev. Osceola, why people pray, and why they hold prayer meetings. "We hold prayer meetings to pray for the sick, the shut in (sick), for healing, for better health, better understanding, those who want to get baptized (converted) and to keep people closer to Christ," he said. "We come together and pray to bring us (community) more together and near. There is more power and strength when we assemble together," he continued. "In the old days we prayed more. We farmers prayed for rain and feared God more. We also had more faith. We would go from house to house praying. We pray to be saved. We pray to keep Satan away and keep in touch with God. Daniel was thrown in the lion's den and they prayed for him three times a day."

"Have women always prayed publicly as they do in church and in prayer meetings?" I asked. "And are these prayer meetings similar to the way in which secret doctors pray for healing?"

"Oh yea!" he exclaimed. "They (secret doctors) once healed in church. God give them (secret doctors) that power to do healing. Some men and women were like prophets. They prophesied. Like everything else, people moving away from old ways and traditions. Yes, women have always prayed. In Titus, Galatians and Timothy they prayed at day and night prayer meetings. And they (women) would give their house to hold prayer meetings," he added.[3]

I also posed the same questions to a Mother of a local Black church. She said, "Oh, we believed in prayer more in olden days. We pray to give thanks, to ask for healing and for self expression. But the same words we said then, we asking the same word now. We must have faith and trust so prayer will be answered. We use to pray every week for rain when I was young. It was always in the morning on a weekday and it was always at church. The prayers always thank God for what God has done, what God can do, and ask God if able to protect and guide us."[4]

Sacrifice and prayer are often said in the same breath. In Yoruba "ebo (sacrifice) means to worship" (Oduyoye 1971, 45). In the African-American context, in order to attain harmony with the universe, a person has to sacrifice by praying and worshiping to appease the Divine and society. On another level, Tylor defines sacrifice as the "gift-theory," a gift made to a deity in exchange for a favor (1920, 376). So it is with the treaters in Louisiana; tokens of gratitude rendered to treaters are actually sacrifices to the Trinity for granting them their petitions. Prayer as a treatment element is not a new healing concept. Within the religious healing phenomenon of these, as well as other, rural African Americans, prayer is a major means of healing (Heyer 1979).

EXAMINATION OF PRAYERS

I observed that the method of prayer in the healing ritual among this research population almost always began with "Oh Father," "Almighty God," or some other reference to God or Jesus. I thought it interesting that God and Jesus were summoned rather than the Holy Spirit, because the Holy Spirit is often the one that appears in visions, dreams, etc. The Holy Spirit is also acknowledged as the source that provides knowledge and wisdom regarding plants, solutions to a particular patient's problem, etc. I felt this defined the relationship with God as more formal and specialized. On the other hand, the relationship with the Holy Spirit, although equally important, is more personal and informal. The role of the Holy Spirit is to act as a messenger, the intermediary between the treaters and God. The Holy Spirit is the deity that relates the "calling" of persons to the treating profession, and it is the deity that comes to the treaters in dreams and visions. The Holy Spirit is also the one who "shows" the treaters certain plants that are good as tea medicine. The Holy Spirit is a regular friend; God and Jesus are special friends. Mbiti (1970) points out that in the African tradition, people communicate directly with God through prayer.

The prayer tradition of African Americans in healing rituals and prayer meetings are simple requests asking God to help with life's basic needs—health, strength, courage, blessings for family, community, etc. There is nothing long and drawn out about these secret doctors' prayers. They last a minute or two. The prayers which take place in prayer meetings are longer. Prayer and prayer incantations in the context of healing rituals and such prayers as those said at prayer meetings are both "magical and religious. . . . Prayer tends very strongly to be magical because of the basic magical coloration of all human symbolic speech and thought" (O'Keefe 1982, 229). Orisons, Catholic prayers said to various saints in the Voodoo tradition in Haiti are in a similar manner—said as amuletic incantations (Metraux 1972, 309).

The kinds of prayers said by individual folk doctors differ. It depends on whether one has a Catholic or Protestant orientation. Although some of the secret prayers are Catholic prayers, this does not necessarily mean that the

individual is Catholic. Formalized Catholic prayers, especially for group praying and those designed to produce altered states of consciousness, such as
praying on prayer beads and the Jesus prayer, influenced the healing ritual
prayer tradition.

The sorts of prayers that are the repertoire of a folk doctor are based on an
oral tradition of the individual's family. For example, Tee Begbe is Baptist,
but most of the prayers he says for healing are Catholic prayers. He says these
prayers because they have been a tradition of secret doctors in his family for
three generations before him. This can be explained by looking at the religious
history of Louisiana. Catholicism was the religion for Blacks and Whites in
Louisiana until the early 1800s. The enslaved African may have brought their
own prayers with them, but due to the circumstances surrounding forced
Christianization of the African, they learned to substitute or replace a Christian prayer, whether verbal or meditative, for a familiar African invocation—
again to camouflage or to make their magicomedical and magicoreligious actions acceptable or at least tolerated.

This careful guarding of the ritual tradition among folk doctors is another
way of preserving structure and order. Knowing how to pray and what to say
in prayer rituals is learned behavior (Mitchell 1986). Prayer content and the
spirituality associated with prayer derive from the African-Americans' experience of oppression and hope for a better tomorrow. The Black prayer tradition then grew out of a need to personalize a relationship with God, a
supernatural being who would be their salvation (Rawick 1972). Most of the
magic (I prefer mysticism) associated with prayer language, just as most of the
theological concepts of religious fervor of the African American, is based on
the Old Testament. However, the New Testament scriptures and the life of
Jesus as a prophet is also important. Scriptures in the New Testament provide
secret doctors with justification for what they do.

Glick (1967, 34) proposes that in any ethnographic study of traditional medicine, the researcher should be concerned with the "people's ideas about loci
of power," and "in their ways of controlling it." "Answers," he continued, "to
questions about locus and control correspond to what are ordinarily signified
by the terms diagnosis and treatment." In rural southwest Louisiana people
believe that God, good spirits, evil spirits, and the devil (Satan) are powerful
agents, and they are responsible for causing illness. God, however, has Supreme power and works through servants—the minister and the secret doctor—to treat illness. Hence, these servants of God utilize prayer and the power
of the supernatural as instruments to treat.

Prayer and faith are essential to the healing ritual, but how one comes into
the profession is equally important and is a deciding factor about the person's
sincerity. Despite the often condescending descriptions of early African-
American beliefs and practices, characterized as "quackery and charlatans,"
data from early sources offer some enlightenment of cultural continuity in
religious beliefs, especially as it relates to the supernatural—visions and

dreams. These data indicate that Black folk doctors have long credited their knowledge about medicine as "a gift from God." Their call to the folk doctor profession parallels that of other Blacks called to the ministry of the Gospel. Their call is often preceded by a dream or vision (Cobb 1851; Postell 1951; Rawick 1972).

Prayer, sacrifice, and worship are not enough within themselves to bring about cures. Faith plays a very important part in affecting the cure. Clients must have faith in God, in the secret doctors and their remedies, and in themselves. To a large degree, the practitioner must be able to strengthen the patient's faith. It is the patient's faith in the healing procedure that will cure, not the procedure (Puckett 1926, 301).

It is important to understand these African-American religious beliefs if we are to understand their beliefs about illness—its causes and cures. Illnesses, by their definition, cannot be cured by medicine alone. There must be help from God and community. African-American ethnomedical beliefs are camouflaged. They are Christians, so it is difficult to get an explanation that is void of Christian dogma. It is also difficult to isolate and say precisely what is attributable to their African, European, or Native American heritage; one can only speculate.

NOTES

1. Folklore Collection #117, Folklore Archives, University of Southwestern Louisiana, Lafayette.

2. The chairman opened the meeting with, "any heart desire tonight." Sister Vensen began with the Lord's Prayer, then proceeded with:

I bow down tonight because you say that every knee must bow and every tongue must confess. And I am bowing tonight to confess to you Jesus. You have been so good. I can thank you all day and all night long.

Oh Lord if you some where round Church to night, I am begging you have mercy Lord.

Now Lord, now, now Lord. [prayer members' response]

Now Lord, if you see anything that look like sin on my heart Jesus I am begging you remove it, so it never rise again. Able you condemn my soul, lead me and guide me Lord. Give me a clear mind Jesus. A better understanding I pray. I want you to talk with me. Don't leave me down here. When I get worry, wipe away my worry.

Now Lord. (members' response)

Those what calling I feel and believe we need you right now. We need you every where we go. We need you on our journey. We need you Lord come by here. I am asking you please in your Holy name go round every sick room tonight Lord. Go round in the hospital remember the poor sick and afflicted one. When they be discouraged please stand by their bedside, ease their pain. Now Lord.

Now Lord (members' response)

Tell them that you is God and beside you there is no other, and you willing. Now Lord. Now Lord. Now, now Lord.

Now Lord. (members' response)

We need you when we riding dangerous highway. We need you at the steering wheel Lord. Lead me and guide me. Oh Lord, Oh Lord, Lordy, Lordy. Thank you Jesus.

Thank you, thank you, thank you. (members' response)

Thank you. Thank you for my last night resting bed. Not only last night but other days, cause we was sleeping an slumbering in our resting bed. Just like dead women, men, and boys and girls. Cause we didn't know nothing for a while. But I feel and believe that you are so good and so kind, you sent one your guiding angels to watch and guide us. Early, early.

Early, early. (members' response)

This morning we don't know how it was done, but we was woken by you Lord to a day we never witness before, and a day that will never return. Jesus.

Jesus. (members' response)

Thank you, thank you Lord. You able me Lord. You able me to put on my shoes. You able me to put on my clothes. You able me to walk around my home and talk with my family. Thank you Jesus. You able me to lie down last night and I was able to get up this morning. Look up on our chairman to night Lord, while he growing old and feeble, please walk with him Lord. Able him. Pray with him. Sing with him. Don't leave him now Heavenly Father. Now Lord.

Now, now Lord. (members' response)

When he get worried rock away his worried mind. Look upon his companion, talk with her, walk with her, don't leave her. Now Lord, now, now Lord. You my rock in the worried land and you my shelter in the time of storm. Thank you for my sisters and brothers. Thank you for my children. Throw your loving arms around them and protect them from all hurt and harm.

Jesus. (members' response)

Lead them and guide them where you have them to go oh Lord don't give them no rest and no peace until they come to know what they must do to be saved, now Lord. Thank you Jesus, oh Jesus don't leave us now Lord, oh Jesus.

Call him up, call him up. (members' response)

Please hear my pray tonight, thank you Jesus. Oh Lord if you some where round Church tonight please come and see about us. Rock away our weary mind Look upon the hospital tonight. You know all about them Lord. Look upon the prison house Lord some of them is in prison Lord. If it be thy holy will Lord we know that you can open prison doors, and we know that you can close them. If it be in your will. Thank you Jesus. Thank you, thank you Lord.

Second Prayer:
   This man began with the Our Father prayer also, then proceeded with:

Here is one of your weak and humble servant. I don't come here for no form and fashion, and neither because I have a head bowed down. But my Father I heard what you said long time ago heavenly Father.

Heavenly Father. (members' response)

You said it be all over. You said every knee must bow and every tongue must confess. Heavenly Father I am bowing and confessing. Heavenly Father, as I come, heavenly Father. I want to first give you thanks. I want to thank you for life, health and strength, heavenly Father.

Thank you, thank you. (members' response)

I want to thank you for last night, Lord as we slept and slumber my Father. We didn't know nothing for ourself and neither for no one else. Father early this morning our eyes fly open we don't know how it was done. We was able to walk with you this morning Lord. You woke us this morning in our right mind and with our health and strength. Heavenly father you able us to get down on our knees. Thank, thank you for giving us one chance.

Thank you. (members response)

Heavenly Father I want to thank you for my companion. Give her wisdom, knowledge and understanding. Lead her the right way. Heavenly Father we love to call your name. Your name fill us when we hunger, water us when we thirsty. Your name will make us walk right. Your name will make us talk right, will make us pray right, will make us sing right.

Help us Holy Spirit. (members' response)

Your name is a mother for the motherless, father for the fatherless, your name is every thing we need Father. Your name is a doctor. Your name is lawyer. Oh please have mercy, we need you in our home. We need you when we traveling a dangerous highway. We need you when things are going right, and when things are going wrong.

We need you. (members' response)

Heavenly Father remember the sick and afflicted every where heavenly Father. Someone is laying in pain all over their body. Heavenly Father tell them not to give up, my Father. Because you is God and there is no other God beside you my Father heavenly Father.

Heavenly Father. (members' response)

Remember Brother Oscar tonight my Father. Lord you know all about him my Father. Heavenly Father tell him you is God and there is no other God my Father. Heavenly Father if you judge him for one thing you can judge for all things.

Yes, Yes. (members response)

Heavenly Father remember Sister Elsie right now my Father Heavenly Father go round her home, touch her family, tell them hasn't been a better time, no other time, heavenly Father. It's getting late and the sun is going down.

Heavenly Father. (members' response)

Remember Brother Zack right now Father. He is a long way from home Father. Heavenly Father. You know his condition, heavenly Father. Tell him not to give up my Father. The doctors tried every thing they could. Tell him you is God my Father. Tell him you is a doctor. Tell him you make the deaf hear, and you make the dumb talk. Lord we know you is able Father to do all things.

You able. (members' response)

Father look down on my sister-in-law. Heavenly Father you know all about her heavenly Father. You know what she is going through. Tell her to trust in your name. Heavenly Father. Tell her your name will make her walk right, talk right. When I walk into my room for the last time ain't got to pray no more.

3. Interview with Rev. Osceola, July 20, 1990, Southwest, Louisiana.

4. Interview with Sister Mother, February 16, 1990, Southwest, Louisiana.

7

Ritual Artifacts

The works of Baker (1980), Deetz (1977), Edwards (1976–1980), Handler 1978, Holloway (1990), Thompson (1984), and Vlach (1978), address the idea of cultural continuity in African-American material culture (such as quilts, foods, architectural design, ritual objects, grave decoration, etc.). This chapter shows the African cultural connection in the folk medicine tradition by examining the protective and curing amulets. My aim is to take a closer comparative look at some aspects of West African, and particularly Congolese, religious thoughts and artifacts and African-American folk medicine in rural Louisiana to determine similarities as a means of validating the culture, its origins, and its religious base.

Although I am not specifically trying to prove that Africanisms survive, I believe some early social scientists' views that traits of African culture could not be found among African Americans in the United States is the basis for the misinterpretation of the African-American folk medicoreligious system. We will probably never fully know, nor understand, the significance of many of these amulets (ritual artifacts) and their uses; however, we can offer speculative guesses. This aspect of the African-American culture has been poorly documented or simply ignored as having very little relevance. Some historical sources (such as plantation diaries, missionary journals), mention these amulets. These documents, however, treat the subject very insignificantly. An example of one observation made regarding enslaved Africans' early use of these healing ritual artifacts follows: "Their superstitions are inseparably mixed with despotism, for they all live under the suzerainty of absolute chiefs. They have

Figure 7.1
Single-Knot String Amulet

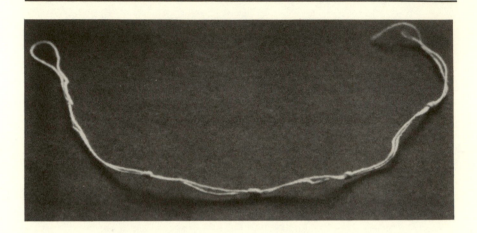

idols or talismans which they venerate and consult, but they soon enough throw them away or burn them" (Robin 1966, 235).

Part of the scarcity of material on the subject is due to the secrecy and sacredness of this tradition. Perhaps too, there just wasn't any significant interest by the literate society to explore the phenomenon of these ritual artifacts. Furthermore, most sources treat the subject out of context—separately and apart from the religious tradition of the African American—thus confusing the issue.

MEDICINAL AMULETS

I have identified nine healing amulets that are frequently used by secret doctors, all *very* varied.

Of the nine amulets, the *single-knot string* amulet (Figure 7.1) is considered the dominant ritual artifact. It usually is made with cord string and has nine knots tied on it. In most cases it is a part of the healing rituals of the treaters and is commonly prescribed for children and adults. The single string amulet can be made to be worn around the waist, across the chest (the string fits over one shoulder and under the opposite arm), the wrist, the ankle, or the neck, depending on what area of the body is afflicted. The common colors are white, red, and black.

The red is used for women of childbearing age who suffer with a history of miscarriages, difficult pregnancies, excessive bleeding after giving birth, and irregular menses. The red string amulet is a specialty of midwives. The white is used for any sex, any age, and any disease. The black is used for young children suffering with worms.

Similar uses of amulets made of cloth string with knots were made by African slaves in the New England region (Piersen 1988). And this single-knot string amulet is used in a similar manner as the cord amulet found in African Independent Churches in Soweto (West 1975). Although there is no genetic tie between Soweto and Louisiana, the Soweto example may hint at an explanation for Louisiana. Also the practices and the beliefs associated with illness in Soweto are very similar to that of Louisiana. Both have African heritage and have contemporary Christian religious beliefs and practices that are a result of syncretism, although different social situations played a part in bringing about the syncretism.

The Bambara, a West African ethnic group and the heritage of many Louisianans, were devout animists and believed very strongly in the use of amulets in healing rituals. One healing amulet they make is a Tafo. It is a cotton cord with knots tied at various intervals very much like the single string amulet (Imperato 1977).

The *multi-knot string* amulet (Figure 7.2) is made with white cord string only and is not very widely used. It is a single white string with a second string tied in multiple knots (macrame fashion) in a complex way forming an intricate design in the center of the original string. The macrame design of the string is almond shaped and about the size of a large almond. It is considered very powerful and is worn around the waist only. According to one folk doctor, the multiple center knots represent every organ and bone in an individual's body. It is commonly prescribed for adults only, and those who suffer with multiple problems (bad luck, bad back, arthritis, worrying, etc.).

The *root necklace* amulet is common among folk doctors whose primary clientele are infants. It is primarily for teething and fever type afflictions in infants and children. It is nine joints of the roots of the mylo herb strung on a white cord string with knots intercepting. It is worn only around the neck.

The *prayer bead necklace* amulet is mainly used for protection and to encourage patients to pray. It is an unspecified number of Job's Tears seeds strung on a white string with knots intercepting each seed. It is worn around the neck. Some people also make rosary beads with these.

Another prayer motivation amulet is the *prayer cloth* (Figure 7.3). It is mainly prescribed for adult men or women, and it is used for protection and healing purposes. It is considered quite powerful. The prayer cloth is always made with red cloth containing various elements, including herb stems forming a cross. It is a one and a half by one and a half inch material element tightly stitched together. The stitching does not appear to have a consistent form. However, I saw two prayer cloths made by the same treater, for the same patient, who was being treated for the same ailment. Both were stitched

Figure 7.2
Multi-Knot String Amulet

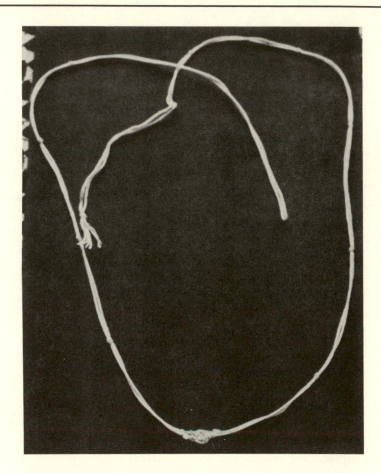

differently. The first, which was octagon shaped, was stitched together to hold several folds of the cloth. The second was stitched only around the edges of the cloth, was folded only once, and it was more of a square shape.

Unlike the string amulets, the prayer cloth is never prepared in the presence of a patient. The ritual associated with its preparation, as well as all of its contents, remains secret. These restrictions are not totally uncommon in traditional healing practices (Hand 1980, 11).

The prayer cloth can also be referred to as a compound amulet. A compound amulet is one that is made of combined protective elements (Hildburgh 1951, 213). What is consistent about the prayer cloth is its color red and the enclusion of plant parts and other elements.

The *Biblical scroll* amulet has scripture headings (chapter and verses from

Figure 7.3
Prayer Cloth

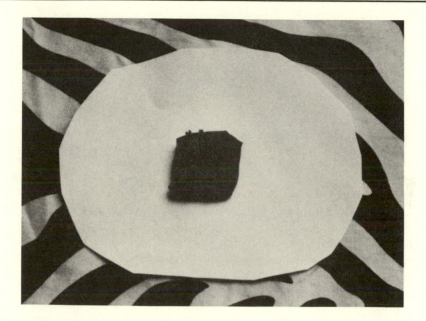

the Bible) on a strip of brown paper bag. It is mainly for adults suffering with afflictions of the limbs (sores, swelling, burns, poor circulation, etc.).

Another kind of amulet used by the Bambara is a type that consists of verses of the Koran written on a bit of paper with names of genies, angels, and formulas. This is then sewn together and worn by the patient. This type of amulet is very similar to one that is found among this research population.

The *walking cane* is a typical dual function material object which serves as an amulet. It is both utilitarian art as well as religious artifact (Vlach 1978, 29, 42). It is used as an amulet, as well as a health aid—to assist with walking.

The cane is carved by its owner (a secret doctor) who believes in the healing and magical powers of plants. The motif on the cane is characteristic of early African-American wood carving art forms, in that an animal motif is carved on it. In one case I saw, a snake's image is curled around the staff.

Beliefs that snakes are satanical and symbolize evil are very prevalent in this community. The metaphorical meaning is that the folk doctor has control, or is in control, of the evil forces that interfere with health and well-being.

Religious lithography (the size of a playing card), images of saints and saintly statues, is another amulet used by several of the secret doctors in this study. Religious lithography, whose function is amuletic, dates back to the middle ages (Lange 1974). It serves a similar purpose in southwest Louisiana as it did in Europe—to protect from disease or other misfortunes. The most common religious lithograph images utilized are those of the Virgin Mary, Saint Michael, and Saint Joseph. It is carried in a person's pocket, wallet, purse, or on their person.

The *silver coin* (usually a dime) amulet necklace, bracelet, or anklet, is not so popular now, but it was fairly popular in recent times. One secret doctor in particular still frequently makes it. The silver coin is pierced and strung on a white cord string. It is usually worn around ankles, the waist, and necks by adults, but I have seen them on babies and small children as well. Its function is mainly protective.

STRUCTURE AND FUNCTION OF AMULETS

A definition of amulets offered by Bonner (1950, 26) may prove helpful at this point. "An amulet is any object which by its contact or its close proximity to the person who owns it, or to any possession of his, exerts power for his good, either by keeping evil from him and his property, or by endowing him with positive advantages."

The belief in the power of amulets to protect the wearer from sickness or harm is widespread in Africa, and that belief was retained by the Africans who came to the Caribbean, South America, Louisiana, and other parts of North America. All amulets in this study are religious in origin, and they all are perishable. They are made of material that is easily destroyed and are not made to last for more than a few months. All the amulets are characteristic of what Nassau (1904, 75) calls "bald fetishism," an object embodied with a spiritual being—in this case the Spirit of God. It is not the fetish that is worshipped, but rather the spirit that is confined within the fetish. Once the spirit leaves the object, it is no longer worshipped.

Hence, the rationale of the treaters that an illness is gone when the string falls off the body; or in the case of Ton Ge Ge, the amulet no longer has its powers after three months, so it is removed from the body and burned. This can also be viewed from the perspective of sympathetic magic (Frazer 1958) and disease transference. Wearing away, however, is the most popular way of disposing of the amulet by patients in southwest Louisiana. The treaters believe that a person can be rid of a disease by transferring the disease to an inanimate object, the string (Hand 1980).

The primary functions of these amulets are curative and preventative—for protection against evil. The power of prayer and the faith of the patient supplements the power of efficacy of the amulets. Historically, amulets have always been thought to have divine attributes (Budge 1930). Unlike the amulets described by Whitten (1973), these rural Louisiana amulets are not associated with evil, nor are they bought from a root doctor or from the treaters. I was told, however, that some form of exchange is expected, so that the amulets can be effective.

The (gift) exchange does not necessarily have to be money, it can be in-kind (such as a crate of yams, okra, or fresh meat from a butchery). Money exchanges range from ten cents to five dollars. Thus strings and prayer cloths are given as a part of the remedy (as medicine), just as a modern doctor prescribes medicine to their patients. As Hildburgh (1951, 231) says, "many things which by our definition are amulets are to their users merely medicines just as simple and as natural in their actions as the decoction of roots and herbs." These amulets have no occult type names such as "mojo," "toby," or the like. They are merely called a string, a prayer cloth, etc.

Plants found as parts of amulets are local medicinal types. Ton Ge Ge is told by the Holy Spirit what "tea medicine plant" is good for treating. These tea medicine plants grow wild in pastures and fields. Numerous sources cite herbs or plants as being used in healing, as well as to ward off evil (Hand 1964; Hyatt 1973).

Another argument based on the power of telepathy is the argument put forth by Gardner, who discusses British talisman and argues that the manner and purpose in which amulets are constructed, where they are constructed, when, and the state of mind of the practitioner when they are constructed, affects the power of the amulet, e.g., morning, midday. "Generally the maker of talismans . . . work is crude and obviously hand-made. . . . The mind of the [talisman]-maker must be concentrated acutely on his work and its purpose. . . . to establish a link with the owner [wearer] and employ the utmost concentration of his will-power to force all the power he can into it [amulet]" (1942:102). Perhaps that is why amulets made in private are considered more powerful than others.

When the treaters were asked why they use a string, none of then could explain why knots were used, why a certain number of knots, why the string was white, etc. It's reasonable that it wasn't ever explained, and it was simply passed on without attention to detail or explanation.

Folk doctors use various combinations of prayer, amulets, and herbs to treat natural illness. Amulets and/or prayer are employed for unnatural causes of illness. If answers to illness or misfortune are not found in one (diagnosis for natural causes), then the other (diagnosis for unnatural causes) is consulted. A person may go to one or more treater, or different types of treaters, including mainstream medicine doctors, seeking a cure or an answer to his or her misfortune.

Amulets which are believed to be embodied with the Holy Spirit, are a manifestation of folk belief. Even more challenging might be to ask why these particular types of amulets are used, and why have these types been chosen for specific purposes. I believe we have already answered "a few" questions; but, probing the psychology underlying folk practices may also offer additional insights into this practice.

Hildburgh (1951, 233) raises the question as to why people continue to use amulets despite the fact that its original function—to produce results that transcend the laws of Nature—is no longer in harmony with the attitudes society currently holds regarding Nature. He concluded that the creation and use of amulets stem from the early instincts of man—the instinct of fear and the craving for protection. In efforts to satisfy those instincts, amulets were created and belief in them was perpetuated. Beliefs in amulets continue to survive, he says, because of the "instinct of childhood credulousness." I argue that infantile conditioning in this community, the instinct of fear and the desire to satisfy that instinct, lies in the faith of the treater and the dynamics of the ritual. The amulet is the result of a person's faith and as such is only one phase of the amuletic process needed to totally satisfy the fear instinct. One is incomplete without the other (ritual and amulet). The whole healing phenomenon is an expression of the rural southwest Louisiana African-American's religiosity—a continual balancing of good and evil.

The dominant amulets, strings, and prayer cloths are made of textile, and they are considered the most powerful of all amulets. Cloth is used cross-culturally as a mode of communication (Schneider and Weiner 1989). In some cultures, such as among the Ewe of Ghana, cloth conveys wealth. The design, color, etc., are intended to communicate knowledge about authority and responsibility. A common thread throughout the history of the African-American tradition is a connection to cloth. One of the most important elements of the African-American material culture tradition is the quilt. The design concepts are believed to be retentions of those found in African textiles (Vlach 1978). This same theory could apply to these material objects of religious fervor—the prayer cloth and knotted strings. Treaters took great pride and patience when making string amulets; they did not simply make a knot. The string had to be turned in an over and under kind of fashion in order to make the "the right kind of knot," as Beedeau patiently demonstrated to me.

Measuring for exactness also seemed to be important "so it could fit right," said Ton Ge Ge who also does the multi-knot string. The strings were never broken by any of the treaters. It was always clipped with scissors; a preference in stitchery art is to cut fabric rather than tear, to avoid shredding or weakening the ends or edges. What was apparent was the concern for quality. Madame Colossi stressed that the "good old time cotton strings" ("good" meaning of top quality) were becoming more difficult to find and if found were often very expensive. Thus these material artifacts demonstrate yet another form of African-American artistic expression.

The idea of tying and knotting in order to link, or bind, forces or as symbols of body parts is found cross-culturally. Ton Ge Ge explained the meaning of the multi-knot string as "representing every bone in a person's body." The "Great Knot," an amulet from Egypt, is thought to represent the bones of the neck that join the head to the body (Howes 1976, 114). Similarly amulets that use tying or binding are considered a means to "arrest a spirit" (Thompson 1984, 120). Although measuring may be considered the least important in relation to the healing phenomenon, it is believed to be a way of determining the physical limitations of disease (Hand 1980, 112).

CROSS-SYMBOLISM

Plants are a very important aspect of religion and medicine in this community. For instance, certain plants are believed to have special powers and are placed in the shape of a cross over doors as amulets to protect households. Within the Christian context, one can say that this practice of placing plants in the form of a cross is an expression of their Christian beliefs. The Christian cross is associated with good and has often been used to overcome evil. It also symbolizes suffering—the "opposite" of that suffering was so that all could have eternal life and peace. A cross could mean to this community just what it symbolizes for eternal life—freedom from sorrow, pain, etc.; after all the foundation of Black theology is based on the Old Testament, the Biblical doctrine which communicates the crucifixion. Using the Christian doctrine to explain, or justify, folk customs is what Mitchell (1975), Cone (1984), and other African-American theologians call the Africanization of Christianity. In addition the number three is involved here—Christ and two of his disciples died on the cross.

Other cross-shaped amulets are not always expressions of faith, nor are they all Christian in origin. In Spain, for example, the Caravaca cross is a modified reproduction of the original Caravaca reliquary in order to coincide with Christianity. According to Hildburgh (1940, 256–57), "a Christian explanation is attached to a form whose origin is pagan . . . in order to win people from pagan beliefs [giving non-Christian practices a Christian explanation], have been a phenomenon common in Christianity's struggle against [non-Christian] rooted religious loyalties.

The pun on the word cross in relation to the literature associated with African-American beliefs linked to illness is that one has been "crossed" (Puckett 1926; Hyatt 1973). This is an example of the theme of opposition, the unharmonious clashing of two forces. Let us refer to the Kongo Cosmogram found in West Africa. The Kongo cruciform (cross) does not symbolize the crucifixion of Christ, however the meaning does overlap. "The Kongo cross refers therefore to the everlasting continuity of all righteous men and women. . . . the crossroads, remains . . . the point of intersection between the ancestors and the living" (Thompson 1984, 108–9). Although the cross may offer no remembrance of African theological beliefs, the folk habit of using it in expressions of religiosity survived (Raboteau 1980, 81).

COLOR SYMBOLISM

When I asked secret doctors if strings, cloth, or the color red had any significance, they replied, "No, it's always been done that way." However, in talking to Maran, she informed me that red cloths are used by "grannies" (midwives) in southwest Louisiana when delivering babies. Also when young children were ill with a respiratory-type illness, grannies would suggest to the mothers to have the child wear red sweaters or red cotton flannel tops "to help them get better." Grannies in this community were usually consulted about childhood illness that were the result of natural causes. In talking with the older female folk doctors, they confirm the use of red. So it seems that red is one of the dominant colors in the community.

In Ardra, a place of Vodu worship in West Africa, the color red is associated with royalty. In most African-American healing practices, it seems as though red is an important color. Thus it is believed the African-American's preference for using red in healing objects, such as amulets, is attributed to their African heritage (Puckett 1926). Similar color patterns and use of certain colors for particular purposes are found in West Africa. Since there is a historical and cultural link between African Americans and West Africa, it is possible then that parallels may be found between the two.

The Ejagham women of West Africa make appliqued cloth coverings called *mbufari*. The *nsibidi* patterning of the cloth reflects status, wit, and proper training determined by the choice of colors—for them, "red equals success in bringing children into the world,' and 'a sign of life;' and white means 'peace' or 'stability of relationship' " (Thompson 1984, 232–33). Restoring health, with the aid of red, can stand to mean restoring life for this community; sickness after all is a form of deterioration—death.

Another dominant color is white. Ton Ge Ge burns a white candle during the treating ritual, and all treaters use white strings. White is a common color used in this community, particularly in relation to the church. The wise female elders of the church wear white every Sunday to designate their status role as female leaders and authorities within the church. White is also worn for baptism and christening. Basically, it is usually associated with purity or some form of spirituality.

INSCRIPTION SYMBOLISM

Another element found in relation to these ritual artifacts are inscriptions. Writing a patient's name on a piece of paper and using it as part of the ritual process is very significant—so are written scriptures. Beedeau and Ton Ge Ge use a piece of paper with the petitioner's name handwritten on it for healing purposes. They say that the patient's birth name has to be written correctly. The married name, nicknames, or a name that has been altered in any way (for instance Wonder, instead of Wonda), is not useful because if inscribed incorrectly the treatment will not work. Names, of course, are symbols of one's individuality. Symbolically, names give the individual power and control of his or her fate.

Similar medicinal amulets are discussed in a study done in Bondoukou,

Ivory Coast, among the Dyula Muslim people who trade for their livelihood. One amulet was "a piece of paper with an inscription from the Qu'ran; any of the ninety-nine names of God, the names of the angels or simply, syllables composed of letters having a special numerical value . . . then fold the paper into thumbnail size and fasten it closed with several winds of cotton string" (Handloff 1982, 186). It was then sewn into a small leather pouch bracelet, or necklace, and worn by persons or attached to objects to protect or heal. Simmons (1971, 57–59) also cites similar "written amulets," in his study in Tonghia, Senegal. The Biblical scroll in this study has similar characteristics and functions. Additionally, some African Americans in Louisiana have Senegalese ancestry.

The written language or inscriptions associated with the design of amulets is an old idea. Wingate (1930) gives a descriptive account of the written charms and Biblical verses found on such an amulet in "The Scroll of Cyprian: An Armenian Family Amulet;" however, this article offers no parallels to that of the Louisiana amulets. The use of inscriptions in amulets could mean, for these people of African heritage, a reflection of indigenous African forms of scrip; "where emblems and ideographs are used as a form of writing to communicate, love, disunity, danger, etc.," (Thompson 1984, 244). Gunther (1905, 154–55) argues that the process of transmission may be responsible for changes of meanings or omissions of certain emblems that were a part of the original amulet. "[T]his change is the exact significance of identical emblems and symbols which we find in different countries and in different times, that renders the study of charms at once so difficult and so fascinating." The notion of names as taboo is very prevalent in magical practices (Frazer 1958).

ENUMERATION SYMBOLISM

Enumeration as a means to ward off evil and supernatural forces is a widespread belief in Italy and Spain. In hopes of confusing or puzzling evil spirits, amulets are often made of several curative components, either in groups or as a single amulet made of two or more amuletic features (Hildburgh 1944). One may rationalize that number patterns are the result of folklore conditioning, just as the trichotomy that exists in American society (Dundes 1975, 224).

The number three, as well as nine, is thought to be complete—nine is considered a perfect and sacred number. It is rarely found in the Bible, but prevails in Egyptian cosmology (Budge 1930). Finally in the case of numbers, secret doctors offer these explanations: Madam Colossi said that it takes nine days for the treatment to "go into effect;" and Beedeau says when he is treating someone, he performs a ritual of praying over his altar at nine in the morning for nine days. Not all cultures use the numbers three and nine in their curative schemes. North American Cherokees use the number four. In order to determine the meaning of number patterns and the difference in therapeutic measures, the geography, culture, and migration must be taken into consideration (Rivers 1924). Even so, the number nine does appear frequently in other African-American communities (Hyatt 1973; Snow 1977b; Webb 1971).

RITUAL AESTHETICS

Some of these healing rituals and altars can be quite elaborate. No two rituals are the same. The way they are carried out depends on the creativity and performance style of each individual healing artist, and a ritual can last from five minutes to an hour or longer.

Patients are impressed with the aesthetics of rituals. The communication process that transpires between the secret doctor and the supernatural powers in the presence of the patient is very important. The beauty and creativity one embellishes these rituals with affects the healing process. The amulet serves as a reminder, a token of that sacredness, divine experience, and a reassurance that protection is with them. This experience to a large degree is psychological.

These rituals are more than just a dramatic show. They are deeply ingrained in a religious ideology that transcends Christian influences. One can conclude that ritual experiences serve as a form of solace for what the psyche remembers. The unexplainable illness is by far the most profound experience for a member of this community. Patients treat such illnesses as delicate and sacred. In most cases, people rely on the wisdom and guidance of secret doctors for a cure or protection from further danger.

In another example, one folk healer shows the changing times of southern culture and the struggle for equality by exhibiting religious lithography and other photo images, such as that of three deceased prophets who influenced social relations in contemporary Black culture—Martin L. King, Jr. and the Kennedy brothers. He (the folk doctor) utilizes an altar for healing purposes with the symbols of power he worships—the religious deities and ancestors. On this altar also lie letters and pictures of clients.

Class distinctions and age often determine the elaborateness and timeliness of a healing ritual. If a person is a farmer, or elderly, then he or she has more time to devote to their craft. The magical aspects appear to be popular among the working and lower class (but it is not exclusively within these classes). These people are less assimilated into mainstream society than a middle- or upper-class person.

Among the upper- and middle-class patients, secret doctors say that you find African Americans who still believe in the healing practices, but they no longer want to wear amulets, particularly amulets that are visible. They find ways to conceal them. Hence some secret doctors do not prescribe them very often anymore.

AMULETS AND SOCIAL CONFLICT

The African-American culture in this region is in a state of transition. Although people continue to practice both Christian and traditional religious traditions, many do not wish to identify with the old ways of acknowledging disease causes and cures. A lack of understanding that these beliefs are culture-based contributes to the confusion. In any case those who are becoming assimilated still resort to old ways of explaining the unexplainable when modern science does not offer a satisfactory explanation.

Ideas about social acceptance are reflected in ritual practices. Some secret doctors specifically stress Christian prayers, and some older secret doctors said talking to God (saying invocations or ritual formulas/proverbs) is acceptable in ritual healing.

Some contemporary patients reject traditional healing methods. They say some elements of healing rituals are incompatible with Christianity (for example, the wearing of amulets is considered to be idol worshiping). Thus more people are choosing not to wear them, they do not want to be associated with "backwards thinking" or "idol worshiping." Instead, they prefer a simple prayer ritual. If they are Catholic, they have no problems carrying lithograph photos of saints. Psychologically though, superstitious beliefs and attitudes often associated with curse and hoodoo remain. People sometimes say they don't believe in icons, which suggest danger or evil, but if they actually encounter superstitious signs, they become skeptical. They would not cross, for instance, a doorway lined with cornmeal. A worldview about the supernatural is deeply imbedded in their psyche and will take more than a simple statement as "backwards thinking," or "idol worshiping" to change traditional beliefs.

Cornmeal is an important aspect of rituals in rural Louisiana. It is often sprinkled across doorways and pathways to symbolize that someone is attempting to bring turmoil or harm to a person or family. If observed at these points, the potential victim avoids these pathways. These beliefs could be related to Papa Legba. Papa Legba, the God of crossroads, survived in Haitian religious practices well into the nineteenth century in early forms of voodoo religious rituals in Louisiana. Salt is also used for similar purposes. One legend of a local community states that salt was sprinkled in a church yard to "cause bitterness and divide the congregation." In Haiti in 1983 I also observed that "maze (cornmeal)" was used to make ve ve signs for the Voodoo ceremonies there. And Puckett (1926, 223) cites a similar example of cornmeal being sprinkled in some form of design in crosspaths among other African-American populations in his study.

There seems to be parallels or borrowing in folk medical traditions between the contemporary African Americans and Native Americans. Paredes, who has done oral history work among the Poarch Creeks in Alabama, claims that Blacks and Native Americans who live in close proximity to each other utilize folk doctors from each others community. The surviving herbal remedies do not appear to be "demonstrably distinctly Indian."

Other areas where parallels exist, or where borrowing may have occurred, are the use of the number nine in ritual healing practices, for example. The Creek Indians use the number nine when constructing a similar healing amulet necklace for teething pain in children as the African Americans in this study do. The Creeks make their necklaces with nine shirt buttons, or nine hog's teeth, or nine beads from the root of the treadsash briar (*Solanum carolinianum*). The research group used nine root joints of the mylo plant to make their amulet necklaces for teething problems. Another example of cultural parallels is the belief that a person who has never seen his or her father has the power to cure thrush by blowing into the mouth of a baby three times. Creeks, as well as African Americans, believe in this remedy (Paredes 1987).

Cultural integration may have taken place between Native Americans and African Americans in ideas about the use of colors and their meanings. Among Louisiana Indians, the color red is used for medicinal practices and is thought to be powerful and the source of life. Among Louisiana Native Americans, red flannel bags filled with herbs were often carried by a sick person as an amulet (Kniffen 1987).

8

Medical Ethnobotany of African Americans

Ethnobotany is the study of plants in a particular culture, and how people in that culture interact with the plants (Ford 1978). My approach to the study of the medical ethnobotany of this population is similar to the approach Messer (1978) used. I was particularly interested in the therapeutic validity of the plants and the cultural beliefs associated with plants and health. Early forms of mainstream medicine had its beginning in the use of herbs or herb properties in patent medicines (Long 1993).[1] I gathered qualitative data for this chapter by observing the ways medicinal plants were used—how folk doctors collected them and how they identified them. I also participated in collecting and utilizing some of the herbs. In addition, I conducted interviews with those known to use medicinal plants in treating.

Most medicinal plants in this study were found in swamps and woods. Some were domestic and could be found in backyards as part of the landscape or in pastures and fields. Those herbs that were found in the pastures and fields were commonly known to locals who relied on herbs for curing benefits; they were the more popular herbs. Medicinal plants found in the swamps and woods were mainly used by secret doctors. Secret doctors took care in gathering these plants and seemed to recognize them by sight more quickly than they could identify them by name. Their identifications and description of uses, were accurate and corresponded to scientific descriptions.

Though there are medical options open to this African-American population, many people still rely on the herbal knowledge and cures of the area. Native medicinal remedies are especially popular with children, women, and older people. Most parents still take their children to secret doctors for childhood diseases such as worms, thrush, teething problems, chicken pox, and measles. Many parents visit secret doctors because they say modern medicine makes the ailment worse and has a smothering effect on children, as in the case of colic.

In most cases, medicinal plants are used as teas or poultices. Others have religious significance. For special problems, some medicinal plants are combined with substances, such as antiseptic, olive oil, whiskey, or vinegar and made into a "tea medicine." Secret doctors charged a small fee for special made tea medicines. One treater charged as high as $15.00 for a half pint of tea medicine he prescribed for heart trouble and nerves. The contents of the tea medicine were unavailable.

CLASSIFICATION OF PLANTS

In this study the plants are classified as teas for (1) infant's and children's sicknesses; (2) women's problems; (3) miscellaneous illnesses, and (4) culinary purposes. Some plants also serve multiple purposes. For example, farmers depend on some plants, such as the sweet potato/yam, for subsistence. The yam is used as food and has medicinal value. One traditional plant, the palmetto, a common plant, had many uses among African Americans. As late as 1908, African Americans continued to utilize the palmetto leaf in constructing their houses (Singleton 1990). The palmetto leaf has also been used in African American coil basket making (Davis 1976). Its leaves were once popularly used locally to make roofs of homes and other buildings.[2] Smaller parts of the palm are placed over doorways to ward off evil, and the root is used to make a tea. There are certain plants that are believed to be taboo. Corn is one of them. Women who are pregnant or are nursing mothers are forbidden to eat it because it is heavy and said to cause medical complications.

PLANT IDENTIFICATION

Most plants are identified through the observation of shapes of the leaves, stems, and color of plants. Some plants that are visibly similar to others are verified by smell. One secret doctor took part of the plant root and rubbed it until an aroma escaped, thus verifying he had the right plant. Plants are also identified according to the part of the plant used, for example, red oak bark, snake root. If leaves were the only parts of the plant used for medicinal purposes, then they are called a tea, for example, mamou tea, sassafras tea.

Roots and barks are reserved for making tea medicines. Tea medicine is a strong liquid mixture made of more than one herb, in large quantities and stored, and taken with directions, such as "three fingers wide" (about a half cup), three times a day. If a plant has a Native American origin, or perhaps was introduced by a Native American to the secret doctor, or has some other association with Native Americans, then the plants are referred to as Indian plants or "my Indian grandmother told me about that plant." Native American women were often the ones cited as the persons who passed on the medicinal plant knowledge.

PLANTS AS FOOD

Corn, sweet potatoes/yams, okra, and rice are main staples for this region. Not only was corn a food staple, but the corn shuck was also popular as a tea. Foods prepared with cornmeal are well-liked as breakfast items. Common breakfast foods made of corn, couch couch and milk[3] or corn bread and milk, are eaten by many rural African Americans in this region.

The sweet potato/yam is especially important to the region as a food stuff for nutrition and for economic reasons. African Americans have a special connection with the yam—it originated in West Africa (Grime 1976). According to Grime's study, okra and blackeyed peas also originated in West Africa. The sweet potato/yam is such an important crop for the region, the locals celebrate it at an annual harvest festival called the Yambilee. The yam/sweet potato is also said to have a laxative effect; it is recommended to regulate the bowels as well as for clear skin. Many other plants cited in this study were mentioned in early investigations identifying plants, shrubs, and trees of the Confederate states that were useful for medicinal, economical, and religious purposes (Porcher 1863).

Ford (1978, 45) argues that unless scholars begin to study "societies that are in the process of change, or that have become westernized," then ethnobotany will become only a literary tradition and an important cultural history will become lost. Ford further points out that environmental variables contribute to change between humans and nature. In the case of southwest Louisiana, sex roles have changed because more women are working away from the farm. Further, environmental hazards, such as pesticides, forbid, in some cases, the gathering of native plants. The altering conditions of the woods and swamps are other environmental variables contributing to change. Large slaughterhouses now provide the fresh meat which individuals once went to the local woods and swamps to obtain; so fewer people are frequenting these spots. As a result, due to the overgrowth of grass, shrubs, trees, etc., it is more difficult to access these woody areas. Japanese plum and catnip tea, for example, now replace certain traditional herbs which were used for the same or similar reasons. Two folk doctors I spoke to had read herb books and recommended new herbs from these books for old ills.

PLANT NAMES

All the plants have at least one name; in some cases they have two. Some plants are named because it is known to cure a certain ailment, for instance, the toothache tree. In some cases, plants are named according to the way they look. The "x" vine is an example. This plant has an x in the center of the vine. Other plants are known by their French names, like Monguilier, indicating that this plant was used since the French colonial period and was perhaps very popular then. The plants that are the most popular are usually the French named plants.

Naming of plants is sometimes symbolic. Berlin (1970, 1) argues that there is a "correlation between lexical retention of plant names and cultural signif- icance of the plant segregates to which plant names refer." For instance among this population the muskedine vine is also called a wisdom vine. Older people (whom are said to be wise), especially, use tea made from the vine for virility and other ailments. In a study by Murphree (1965), she con- cluded that folk terminology associated with medicinal plants often described the property or the appearance of the plant. It is not uncommon for distinc- tive ethnic groups to give plants culturally-derived names, based on their use, character, physical appearance, or environment. Tewa Indians and Santo Domingo's plant names are also culturally derived (Colon 1976–1977; Rob- bins 1916).

Two vernacular factors contributed to the difficulty I encountered in looking up data on some of these plants; one difficulty was finding the common names that were used by African Americans and other native groups; another diffi- culty I encountered was that some plants were only commonly known by a Creole French name, which often made it hard for botanists outside of Lou- isiana to identify.[4]

RELIGION AND PLANTS

Preparing teas or ritual artifacts with certain plants often included magical practices. Cutting nine pieces of a root or vine to make tea medicines or taking three fingers of the tea as a dosage to produce magical effects are popular examples. Other examples of plants as ritual objects are the x plant being used to uncross (remove a hex or curse) and palmetto leaves placed above doorways in the form of a cross to ward off evil and protect households. These examples also characterize the religious connections.

Praying over the medicine while one prepares it is also common. Some plant parts are used as amulets to ward off evil as well as to cure. Tee Begbe used the blackjack vine to make a walking cane as a healing and protective element. It seems as though these medicinal plants are a natural part of the ongoing cosmology of the people. Dreams also played an important part in giving the folk doctors knowledge about plants and their uses.

AVAILABILITY AND CULTURAL CHANGE

The changing sex roles of women contribute to change in the traditional methods of gathering medicinal plants. Women are moving toward work outside the home, so folks now feel a woman's place is not in the woods digging and looking for plants. Environmental hazards are also causing changes in the availability of certain plants. New plants are being introduced, and some native plants are becoming less available; however, some old plants remain popular and plentiful. Those popular plants found near the homes are those this society is especially partial to. People plant and replant them to assure their survival.

There seems to be a rebirth of the use of herbs; maybe this has to do with the renaissance of alternative medicine. What I found interesting with herbal use, was a tendency, especially among younger people (under the age of 50), to prefer "store bought" herbs versus native herbs. I believe this preference is due to the desire for social acceptance by the broader community, and store bought herbs is a way to avoid conflicts associated with prescribing medicines/herbs that are unfamiliar to mainstream society. A secret doctor might tell a patient "go to the health food store and ask what herb is good for kidney trouble," or they might recommend a herb, adding "you can buy it at the health food store."

Today, many female secret doctors avoid going into woody areas, in contrast to several years ago when women went into woods and swamps to gather herbs just as frequently as men did. Women now claim they avoid these areas because they fear snakes and other poisonous or dangerous creatures. Additionally, they say they are more comfortable inside their homes with the convenience of air conditioners.

Other instances where the issue of store bought herbs was a concern was that of a female folk doctor who always recommends these herbs. Her rationale is that the store bought herbs work just as well as the native ones, "there is no difference." Furthermore, she seems to respect information she reads in herbal books and the advice she gets from persons in health food stores. She identified one person in a health food store as "doctor." When I asked was the person a medical doctor she said "No." So I said, "Oh, he's a treater!" She responded, "No, I don't think so, but he must be some kind of doctor since he knows so much about herbs." Among most secret doctors fifty and above however, very strong and firm beliefs in tradition exist; hence, traditional herbs and methods of practicing are maintained.

Seed jewelry is not a new idea. Seeds, and other items such as bone, have been used in jewelry to adorn the body and for protection against evil and disease since the fifth dynasty in Egypt (Moore 1982). This tradition of using plant parts in healing rituals for curing purposes survives today in this rural community. One such plant is Job's Tears. The seeds are used to make prayer beads, as well as amulet necklaces for protection and curing purposes.

Cousan Nom stated that the red seeds of the Mamou plant, in addition to being an excellent tea for colds and influenza-related illnesses, were once made as necklaces for women. This was a common practice in other areas of Louisiana as well.[5]

PLANT KNOWLEDGE

Perhaps the greatest influence the Native Americans had on the African-American culture is through the passing on of their oral plant knowledge. Several of the people I interviewed credited their Native American ancestry for their knowledge about herbal remedies. In addition to racial intermixing, medical ethnobotany displays the strongest influence of African American and Native American intermingling. Among the early Creeks, for example, cedar leaves, oak, and cane were among the plants used in teas taken by the men in preparation for the annual Busk ceremony (Gatschet 1884). One interviewee in this study cited cane root as a good medicinal herb. Other persons in the community value cedar trees as part of the home yard landscape, and additionally as a good luck tree.

Besides the influence of plant knowledge, intercultural exchanges between the Native American and African American took place in other aspects. The design and construction of the drum of the Bayou Lacomb Choctaw, for example, is believed to have been influenced by the African American (Bushnell 1909). The Louisiana Choctaws also have a legend related to how their medicine doctors acquired knowledge about herbs. When a child is three or four years old, it is often sick and runs away from home where he meets Kwano-kasha, a little spirit, who leads the child to another dwelling place. They then meet three other spirits, very old, who:

Approaching the child the first offers it a knife; the second a bunch of herbs, all poisonous; the third a bunch of herbs yielding good medicine. Now, if the child accepts the knife he is certain to become a bad man, and may even kill his friends. If he takes the bunch of poisonous herbs he will never be able to cure or otherwise help others; but if he waits and accepts the good herbs, then he is destined to become a great doctor and an important and influential man of his tribe, and to have the confidence of all his people. In this event Kwanoka'sha and the three old spirits tell him how to make use of the herbs—the secrets of making medicines of the roots and leaves and of curing and treating various fevers and pains. The child remains with the spirits three days, after which he returns to this home but does not tell where he has been or what he has seen and heard. Not until the child has become a man will he make use of the knowledge gained from the spirits, but never will he reveal to others how it was acquired (Bushnell 1909, 30–31).

Perhaps fusion occurred between these Choctaw and African Americans. African Americans in Louisiana believe that knowledge about herbs and their uses come from the "Holy Spirit," and any person who does not receive their knowledge from the Holy Spirit, and abuses people under the guise of a old secret doctor, will be punished. They believe that people who do not interact with the Holy Spirit are working for an evil spirit, Satan. African Americans believe that a good doctor is someone who has faith, endurance, is prayerful, and "waits" on answers from God. Although a child may have visions or dreams usually, it is not until he or she is an adult that he or she becomes a full-time practitioner—although the "gift" was received in childhood.

Patricia Rickles cites an interesting account which exemplifies the many oral history narratives I encountered pertaining to Red/Black mixtures and inherited ethnobotany knowledge. She reports:

One Black family from the Carencro (Louisiana) area has handed down the story of a female ancestor who was Atakapas Indian. This women was so skilled in finding, preparing and administering medicinal herbs. . . . Once each year she went on a secret trip into the wilderness to meet with other Indians and gather herbs for her healing work. (1975, 147)

Another concern of this research was to try and determine what knowledge about plants, and what specific plants used by this community, originated in West Africa. To this date that has been difficult (some exceptions are the yam/sweet potato, okra, and blackeyed peas). The yam is not necessarily medicinal, but it is often eaten for health reasons. Blackeyed peas have religious significance. For good fortune throughout a new year, African Americans eat blackeye peas on New Years day. And the okra is an all time favorite vegetable staple, eaten with rice or in gumbos.

Regarding a plant's African origin, I discovered that knowledge is limited. It is difficult to ascertain specifically whether the plant knowledge of secret doctors is credited mostly to their African heritage or to their Native American encounter. Harvey (1981, 157) indicates: "The bulk of the material (on African Americans' use of plants) is unsystematically gathered, heavily anecdotal, and was written when expressed anti-Black sentiments and racial slurs were acceptable in what passed for scientific works."

Secret doctors came to Louisiana with knowledge about medicinal plants. Knowledge about new plants was properly acquired by first identifying the plant based on physical appearance, and secondly by testing (trial and error) the plant to determine if its properties were similar to ones previously found in Africa. Just how the early secret doctors went about determining what plants had particular qualities is only speculative. Certainly acknowledging environmental conditions is important. Knowing a certain plant's habitat is important in knowing where and when to search for it. The Louisiana landscape and subtropical climate is not totally unlike the terrain and climatic conditions of tropical Africa.

Several plants that appear in this collection are members of plant families in West Africa. These appear in a study done by Sofowora (1982) on West African medicinal plants. Those West African plant families found in this study are also widely distributed throughout other parts of the world. They are the

Croton, Dioscorea, Orimum, Sambucus, Zea mays, Aristolochia, and Ocimum families. In any case these data clearly indicate that African Americans have a tradition of interacting with the plant world, and that plants are important in health, religion, and other aspects of African-American life.[6] Refer to the Appendix for names and descriptions of plants' commonly used by African Americans in this region.

CONCLUSION

This ethnographic study documents this ethnomedicine tradition as a valid organized medical system because: (1) secret doctors/treaters must meet certain qualifications before becoming treaters; (2) they have an established history of successes; and (3) the ethnomedical system contains a body of knowledge that is based on an oral tradition. Secret doctoring (a local term used to describe the folk medicine practitioners and what they do) survives because of trust, common cultural values and beliefs in the causes of illness, and because it is economically feasible.

The folk medical beliefs and practices of the Louisiana secret doctors are sought by Baptists and Catholics whose theological beliefs are based on orthodox religious doctrines and non-orthodox religious healing customs that are simultaneously practiced. The secret doctors are all Christian men and women who are active in their local churches and whose basic philosophy is that God is supreme, God is the healer, and God does heal.

On the other hand, they offer very little explanation for the non-orthodox religious aspect of what they do. This mainly involves the use of animistic objects (amulets) as part of the remedy in healing rituals. These ritual artifacts (knotted strings, prayer cloths, prayer beads) are credited to their Central African (Congolese) heritage.

Overall, this study shows that this syncretic practice is merely an expression, or extension, of the religiosity of the people. Syncretic in this particular study means a merging or combining of two theologies and methods of worshiping. These people with West African bloodlines continue to carry on a tradition that was the custom of their foreparents. In the African-American cultural tradition, we find what is not retained are the theological explanations for what they do; what is remembered are folk customs.

When Africans adopted Christian beliefs, they incorporated the Christian doctrine with their folk customs to make it seem as though they were true believers of Christianity. The basic elements of Christianity were indeed visible—Christian prayers, the crucifix, Christian saints, etc. However, the wearing of a mask to conceal or defy true character is a common theme throughout the history of African Americans. The hidden meanings in the spirituals is a good example of this (Southern 1971). A similar thread is found behind the veil of folk healing in rural southwest Louisiana where three cosmologies interplay—Christian, African, and Native American perspectives.

Although Christian concepts did not replace the spiritual remembrance of the old medicoreligious traditions, nor destroy the spirituality within, they did offer some protection from hostile tongues of ridicule. Behind the mask of certain African-American Christian churches, folk religious and treating practices survived. Thus prayer, faith, and the power of the Holy Spirit embodied within a material object became the three key Christian elements for the healing rituals.

Beliefs based on the Christian doctrine manifested through objects based on animistic concepts became the foundation for ethnomedical practices in this rural southwest community in Louisiana. The belief in prayer, in plants, in amulets, and in a particular interpretation of the supernatural (characteristic of treating methods) survived.

NOTES

1. Long, Jim. "Patent Medicines," *The Herb Companion* 5 (1993): 48–52.
2. In a 1908 survey of early African-American homes conducted by W.E.B. Dubois he offers this description: "the dwellings of slaves were palmetto huts, built by themselves of stakes and poles, with the palmetto leaf" (Singleton 1990:3).
3. A cereal-type food that is prepared with corn meal and water.
4. A good source of common plant names is King, Lawrence J. "Annotated Bibliography of Studies Relating to the common or Popular Names of Plants," *Plant Lore* 6 (1982):11–16.
5. Folklore Collection #277, Folklore Archives, University of Southwestern Louisiana, Lafayette.
6. Other plants appearing in this study were verified in the following sources: Duke (1985); Everett (1982); Krochmal (1973); Landry (1989); Morton (1981); Taylor and Thomas (1985); and Touchstone (1983).

Appendix: Medical Ethnobotany Plant List

The following is a list of the plants I collected. I give their common name(s), followed by their scientific name, and a general statement about their uses and habitat.

1. Palmetto Root (*Sabal minor*). The root is used as a tonic tea. This plant is found in swamps and marshy areas.
2. Wisdom Vine (muskedine) (*Vitis rotundifolia*). The vine is boiled to make a tea. Muskedine grows wild and is found growing around trees in woody areas. It bears a grape-like fruit, a favorite fruit for locals. Muskedine preserves and homemade wine are other favorite culinary delights. The tea is good for kidney problems and dropsy (fluid retention).
3. Peach Leaves (*Prumus persica*). The leaves are used to make tea for female health problems. It is a domestic plant.
4. Corn Shuck Tea (*Zea mays*). The shuck covering of dry corn is boiled as a tea and taken for influenza and colds. It is a domestic plant.
5. Catnip Tea (*Nepeta cataria*). The leaves are made as a tea for colds and for colic in children. It is a domestic plant.
6. Iron Leaf (ironweed) (*Veronia missurica*). The leaves are used to make a tea for weak bladder. It is found in wooded areas.

7. Tea Grass (teaweed) (*Sida rhombibolia*). This small shrub grass is used to make a tea for fever. It is found in fields and pastures.

8. Snake Root (*Aristolochia serpentaria*). The roots of this plant are boiled and taken as a tea. Its properties are similar to penicillin. It is very good for infections, viruses, and liver and kidney problems. Is found in swamps, wet, woody, and shady areas. It is becoming scarce.

9. Hackberry (tree we already knew) (*Celtis laevigata*). The bark of this tree, found in the woods, is used to make a tea and is cut in a round fashion. It is good for kidney ailments and diabetes.

10. Mayapple (American mandrake) (*Podophyllum peltatum*). The leaves are used to make a tea. It is taken as a purger after taking other herbs to heal. It is a domestic plant.

11. Le Mamou (coral bean) (*Erythrina herbacea*). The root is boiled and the tea is heavily sweetened to make a cough syrup; or it can simply be drunk as a tea. The beans of this plant were once used to make necklaces for women and girls. The tea is good for colds. The herb is found in woods, pastures, and in back yards; it is common and very popular.

12. l'Herbe a Malo (arrowhead) (*Sagittaria platyphylla*). This is a very popular plant for treaters. They cut the roots at its joints (usually in nine pieces) and string them on white cord strings to put around babies' necks for teething problems. Is said to "draw fever" out of babies and to "kill the pain" from teething. It is found in very soggy swamp land.

13. Elderberry (*Sambucus canadensis*). The root is boiled to make a tea. The tea is taken for bladder infections. It is found in woody areas.

14. Indian Turnip (Jack-in-the-pulpit) (*Arisaema triphyllum*). The root is boiled and taken as tea for kidney, liver, and ulcer problems. It is also eaten, but burns the stomach when eaten raw (similar to cayenne pepper). It is found in woody and damp areas.

15. Dogwood Tree (*Cornus florida*). The root is boiled and made into a tea. The tea is good for cleansing and inflammation. It is a domestic plant.

16. Wild Plum (*Prunus americana*). The bark of the wild plum tree is boiled and taken as a tea to treat asthma. It is found in wooded areas.

17. Courtableu Tea (*Catalpa bignonioides*). The bark of the tree is boiled and taken as a tea for purging. The leaves are also boiled to make a dye for clothing. And, at Easter, the leaves are boiled and wrapped around eggs to dye easter eggs. The wood is also considered very strong and has sometimes been used for building. It is found in wooded areas.

18. Camphor Tree (*Cinnamomum camphora*). The leaves and bark are used in teas for colds. It is found in pastures and fields.

19. Bay tree (Lo dee al) (sweet laurel) (*Persea borbonia*). The bark is boiled as a tea for liver problems and colds. Some take the leaves and make a cross over their front doors to ward off evil. The leaves are also popular as a spice. It is found in pastures.

20. Indian Pink/Pink root (worm grass) (*Spigelia marilandica*). Leaves are used to

make a tea for children suffering with worm problems. It is found in pastures and fields.

21. Toothache Tree (prickly ash) (*Zanthoxylum clava-herculis*). The inner bark is used to rub on the gums of adults for toothache. It has a real numbing effect. It is found in pastures and fields.

22. Carencro plant (spice bush) (*Lindera benzoin*). The leaves of this mint tea is used for arteritis. It is combined with corn shuck and sassafras and made into a tea to promote clear skin for children. It is found in pastures and fields.

23. Mamou Potato (Le contaque) (*Smilax rotundifolia*). Boil root bulb of this plant until it becomes a broth mixture and use as a tea for dropsy. It is found in woods and swamps.

24. Garlic (*Allium sativum*). Garlic is placed around the waist in a cloth pouch for worms in children and stomach infections in adults and children. Adults also take it as a tea for cleansing the bowels. It is a domestic plant.

25. Blackjack Vine (*Sagittaria platyphylla*). The vine is boiled as a tea to purify the blood. It is also used to make walking canes (protective) and furniture. It is found in woods and swamps.

26. Red Oak Bark (swamp red oak) (*Quercus shumardii*). The bark is mixed with other herbal plants to make tea medicine for diabetes. It is found in woody areas.

27. Le Monguilier (groundselbush) (*Baccharis halimifolia*). This is a local, extremely popular and effective herb. The leaves and branches are boiled and taken as a tea for colds and fever. It grows wild everywhere (pastures, side of roads, mostly in well-drained places).

28. Sheep Tea (goat plant/goatweed) (*Croton capitatus*). This is another popular plant. The leaves and stems are made into a tea for influenza-type ailments. This tea mixed with ice induces relaxation. It was once easily found growing wild in pastures, but is now becoming scarce.

29. Sassafras (*Sassafris albidum*). The root of this plant is boiled and drunk as a general purpose tea. The tea is good for gallstones, to clear sinuses, and for cleansing the blood. The leaves are mashed and made into the popular gumbo spice—file. It is found in pastures and fields.

30. Baume Tea (Le baume sauvage) (*Monarda punctata L.*). The leaves and stems of this mint-tasting plant are used as a tea for colds. The tea is also given to cure colic and dysentery. It is a common domestic plant.

31. Yam/Sweet Potato (*Dioscorea alata L.*). This tuber food is good to regulate the bowels. It is found in fields.

32. La Basilioue (common basil) (*Ocimum basilicum*). The leaves of this plant are made into a tea and taken as a tonic. It is also used as a culinary spice to flavor gravies. It is a domestic plant.

33. Prayer Seeds (Job's tears) (*Coix lacrym jobi*). The seeds of this plant are used to make prayer necklaces, or rosary beads, for protective purposes. It is domestic, but not very common. Only certain secret doctors grow this plant.

34. Dewberry (*Rubus trivialis*). The leaves and stems of this plant are made into a tea. It is good for bladder infections and edema. It is found in pastures and fields.

References

Abrahams, Roger D., and John F. Szwed. *Afro-American Folk Culture: Part I—North America: An Annotated Bibliography of Materials from North, Central, South America & West Indies*. Philadelphia: Institute for Study of Human Issues, 1978.

Allain, Mathe. "Slave Policies in French Louisiana." *Louisiana History* 21 (1980): 127–137.

Allen, Charles M., and R. Dale Thomas. *Contributions of the Herbarium of Northeast Louisiana University: A Checklist of the Woody Plants of Louisiana*, No. 2. Monroe, La.: Northeast Louisiana University, 1981.

Avery, Byllye Y. "Breathing Life Into Ourselves: The Evolution of the National Black Women's Health Project." In *The Black Women's Health Book: Speaking for Ourselves*, edited by Evelyn C. White, 4–10. Seattle: Seal Press, 1990.

Axelsen, D. E. "Women as Victims of Medical Experimentation: J. Marion Sims' Surgery on Slave Women, 1845–1850." *SAGE* 2, no. 2 (1985): 10–13.

Bacon, Alice Mabel. "Folk Lore Scrap-Book," *Journal of American Folklore* 9–10 (1896–1897): 143–147.

Bacon Alice Mabel, and Leonora Herron. "Conjuring and Conjure-Doctors." In *Mother Wit From the Laughing Barrel: Readings in the Interpretation of Afro-American Folklore*, edited by Alan Dundes, 359–368. Englewood Cliffs, N.J.: Prentice-Hall, Inc., 1973.

Baer, Hans A. "Toward a Systematic Typology of Black Folk Healers." *Phylon: The Atlanta University Review of Race and Culture* 43 (1982): 327–343.

Baer, Hans A., and Merrill Singer. *African-American Religion in the Twentieth Century: Varieties of Protest and Accommodation*. Knoxville: University of Tennessee Press, 1992.

Bair, Barbara, and Susan E. Cayleff. *Wings of Gauze: Women of Color and the Experience of Health and Illness*. Detroit: Wayne State University Press, 1993.

Baker, Vernon. "Archaeological Visibility of Afro-American Culture: An Example from Black Lucy's Garden." In *Archaeological Perspectives on Ethnicity in America: Afro-American and Asian American Culture History*, edited by Robert L. Schuyler, 29–47. New York: Baywood Publishing Co., Inc., 1980.

Barnhart, Joe. "Faith Healers in a Naturalistic Context." *The Humanist* 48, no. 5 (1988): 5–8.

Barrett, Leonard E. *Soul Force: African Heritage in Afro-American Religion*. New York: Anchor Press/Doubleday, 1974.

Barroso, C. "Female Sterilization: Free Choice and Oppression," *Revista de saude publica* 18, no. 2 (1984): 170–180.

Bartels, Charles. "Louisiana Women Add to the Work Force." *Opelousas* (Louisiana) *Daily World*, June 25, 1989, 8.

Bascom, William. "The Relationship of Yoruba Folklore to Divining." *Journal of American Folklore* 56 (1953): 127–131.

———. *Shango in the New World*. Austin, Tex.: African and Afro-American Research Institute, The University of Texas, 1972.

Bassett, Mary T., and Nancy Krieger. "Social Class and Black-White Differences in Breast Cancer Survival." *American Journal of Public Health* 76, no. 12 (1986): 1400–1403.

Bastide, Roger. *African Civilizations in the New World*. Translated by Peter Green. London: C. Hurst & Company, 1971.

———. *The African Religions of Brazil*. Translated by Helen Sebba. Baltimore: The John Hopkins University Press, 1978.

Bell, Michael Edward. "Pattern, Structure and Logic in Afro-American Hoodoo Practices." Ph.D. diss., Indiana University, 1980.

Bell-Scott, Patricia, and B. Guy-Sheftall, eds. "Special Issue: Health." *SAGE* 2, no. 2 (1985): 2–78.

Bergman, Peter. *The Chronological History of the Negro in America*. New York, Evanston, and London: Harper and Row, 1969.

Berlin, Brent, Dennis E. Breedlove, and Robert M. Laughlin. *Lexical Retention and Cultural Significance in Tzeltal-Tzotzil Comparative Ethnobotany*, No. 29. Berkeley: University of California, Language Behavior Research Laboratory, 1970.

Berlin, Ira. *Slaves Without Masters: The Free Negro in the Antebellum South*. 1974 Reprint. New York: Vintage Books, 1976.

Bernstein, Barbara, and Robert Kane. "Physicians' Attitudes Toward Female Patients." *Medical Care* 19, no. 6 (1981): 600–608.

Blake, John B. "Women and Medicine in Ante-Bellum America." *Bulletin of the History of Medicine*, 39, no. 2 (1965): 99–123.

Boles, John. *Black Southerners, 1619–1869*. Lexington, Ky.: The University Press of Kentucky, 1943.

Bonner, Campbell. *Studies in Magical Amulets: Chiefly Greco-Egyptian*. Ann Arbor: The University of Michigan Press, 1950.

Bossu, Captain. *Travels Through that Part of North America Formerly Called Louisiana*, vol. 1. Translated by John Reinhold Foster. London: T. Davies in Ruffel Street, Covent Garden, 1771.

Bourguignon, Erika, and Louanna Pettay. "Spirit Possession, Trance and Cross Cultural Research." In *Symposium on New Approaches of the Study of Religion*, edited by June Helm, 38–49. Proceedings of the 1964 Annual Spring Meeting of the American Ethnological Society. Seattle and London: University of Washington Press.

Boxall, Jean F. "Sayings and Superstitions." *Midwives Chronicle and Nursing Notes* (December 1988): 400.

Brackenridge, Henry Marie. *Views of Louisiana: Together With a Journal of a Voyage up the Missouri River, in 1811.* 1814. Reprint. Chicago: Quadrangle Books, 1962.

Braithwaite, Ronald L., and Sandra E. Taylor, eds. *Health Issues in the Black Community.* San Francisco: Jossey-Bass Publishers, 1992.

Brandon, Elizabeth. " 'Traiteurs' or Folk Doctors in Southwest Louisiana." In *Buying the Wind: Regional Folklore in the United States,* edited by Richard M. Dorson, 261–266. Chicago and London: The University of Chicago Press, 1964.

Brasseaux, Carl A. "Arrival of Acadians From Santo Domingo." *Atakapas Gazette* 10 (1975): 146–150.

———. "The Administration of Slave Regulations in French Louisiana, 1724–1766." *Louisiana History* 21 (1980): 139–158.

Brooks, Evelyn. "The Women's Movement in the Black Baptist Church, 1880–1920." Ph.D. diss., University of Rochester, 1984.

Budge, Sir E. A. Wallis. *Amulets and Superstitions.* London: Oxford University Press, 1930.

Bushnell, David I., Jr. *The Choctaw of Bayou Lacomb St. Tammany Parish Louisiana.* Washington, D.C.: Bureau of American Ethnology, Bulletin 48, Government Printing Office, 1909.

Bushy, A. "Rural United States Women: Traditions and Transitions Affecting Health Care." *Health Care Women International* 11, 4 (1990): 503–513.

Butler, Joseph T., Jr. "The Atakapa Indians: Cannibals of Louisiana." *Louisiana History* 11 (1970): 167–176.

Butler, Melvin Arthur. "African Linguistic Remnants in the Speech of Black Louisianians." *Black Experience: A Southern University Journal* 55 (1969): 45–52.

Campinha-Bacote, Josepha, and Regina J. Allbright. "Ethnomusic Therapy and the Dual-diagnosed African American Client." *Holistic Nursing Practice* 6, no. 3 (1992): 59–63.

Capers, Cynthia Flynn. "Nurses' and Lay African Americans' Views About Behavior." *Western Journal of Nursing Research* 13, no. 1 (1991): 123–135.

Carter, Harold A. *The Prayer Tradition of Black People.* Valley Forge, Pa.: Judson Press, 1976.

Chesnutt, Charles W. "Superstitions and Folklore of the South." In *Mother Wit from the Laughing Barrel: Readings in the Interpretation of Afro-American Folklore,* edited by Alan Dundes, 369–378. Englewood Cliffs, N.J.: Prentice-Hall, Inc., 1973.

Chidsey, Donald Barr. *Louisiana Purchase.* New York: Crow Publishers, Inc., 1972.

Christian, Barbara. "Community and Nature: The Novels of Toni Morrison." *Journal of Ethnic Studies* 7 (1980): 65–78.

———. "The Race for Theory." *Feminist Studies* 14, 1 (1988): 67–79.

Christian, Marcus. *Negro Ironworkers of Louisiana: 1718–1900.* Gretna, La.: Pelican Publishing Company, 1972.

Clarke, Adele. "Subtle Forms of Sterilization Abuse: A Reproductive Rights Analysis."

In *Test-Tube Women: What Future for Motherhood?* edited by Rita Arditti, Renate Duelli Klein, and Shelley Minden. London: Pandora Press, 1984.

Cobb, Henry E., and Thelma Cobb. "Ethnicity and the Louisiana Heritage: Humanistic Considerations." In *Louisiana's Future: Whose Responsibility?*, edited by James Lockett 5–11. Baton Rouge, La.: Southern University, 1977.

Cobb, Joseph B. *Mississippi Scenes: Or Sketches of Southern and Western Life and Adventure*. Philadelphia: A. Hart, Late Carey and Hart, 1851.

Cole, Johnetta B. "Africanisms in the Americas: A Brief History of the Concept." *Anthropology and Humanism Quarterly* 10 (1985): 120–126.

Colliard, Rev. B. "Rummaging Through Old Parish Records: Historical Sketch of the Parish of Opelousas, Louisiana." *St. Louis Catholic Historical Review* 3 (1921): 14–38.

Colon, Sandra Hernandez. "The Traditional Use of Medicinal Plants and Herbs in the Province of Pedernales, Santo Domingo." *Ethnomedicine* 4 (1976–77): 139–166.

Conco, W. Z. "The African Bantu Traditional Practice of Medicine: Some Preliminary Observations." *Social Science and Medicine* 6 (1972): 283–322.

Cone, James H. *For My People: Black Theology and the Black Church*. Maryknoll, N.Y.: Orbis Books, 1984.

Cope, Nancy R., and Howard R. Hall. "The Health Status of Black Women in the U.S.: Implications for Health Psychology and Behavioral Medicine." *SAGE* 2, 2 (1985): 20–24.

Crowe, Charles. "Indians and Blacks in White America." In *Four Centuries of Southern Indians*, edited by Charles Hudson, 148–169. Athens, Ga.: University of Georgia Press, 1975.

Darst, Judith Ward Steinman. "Newspaper Medicine: A Cultural Study of the Colonial South 1730–1770." Ph.D. diss., Tulane University, 1971.

Dart, Henry P. "Editor's Chair." *Louisiana Historical Quarterly* 9 (1926): 286–287.

———. "The Spanish Procedure in Louisiana in 1800 for Licensing Doctors and Surgeons." *Louisiana Historical Quarterly* 14 (1931): 204–206.

———. "The First Cargo of African Slaves for Louisiana, 1718." *Louisiana Historical Quarterly* 14 (1931): 163–171.

Davis, Angela. *Women, Race and Class*. New York: Vintage Books, 1983.

———. "Sick and Tired of Being Sick and Tired: The Politics of Black Women's Health." In *The Black Women's Health Book: Speaking for Ourselves*, edited by Evelyn C. White 18–26. Seattle: Seal Press, 1990.

Davis, G. L. "Afro-American Coil Basketry in Charleston County, South Carolina." In *American Folklife*, edited by Don Yoder, 151–184. Austin: University of Texas Press, 1976.

Davis, John, trans. *Travels in Louisiana and the Floridas in the Year 1802*. New York: I. Riley and Company, 1806.

Davis, John, ed. *Africa from the Point of View of American Negro Scholars*. Dijon, France: Imprimerie Bourguignonne, 1958.

Deetz, James. *In Small Things Forgotten: The Archeology of Early American Life*. Garden City, N.Y.: Anchor Press/Doubleday, 1977.

DeLatte, Carolyn E. "The St. Landry Riot: A Forgotten Incident of Reconstruction Violence." *Louisiana History* 17 (1976): 41–49.

Desdunes, Rodolphe Lucien. *Our People and Our History*. Translated and Edited by

Sister Dorothea Olga McCants. Baton Rouge: Louisiana State University Press, 1937.

DeVille, Winston. *Opelousas: The History of a French and Spanish Military Post in America, 1716–1803.* Cottonport, La.: Polyanthos, 1973.

Dillingham, B. "Indian Women and Indian Health Service Sterilization Practice." *American Indian Journal* 3, no. 1 (1977): 27–28.

Dominguez, Virginia R. *Social Classification in Creole Louisiana.* New Brunswick, N.J.: Rutgers University Press, 1986.

Donald, Henderson H. *The Negro Freedman: Life Conditions of the American Negro in the Early Years After Emancipation.* New York: Henry Schuman, 1952.

Dormon, James H. *The People Called Cajuns: An Introduction to an Ethnohistory.* Lafayette, La.: The Center for Louisiana Studies, University of Southwestern Louisiana, 1983.

Dorson, Richard. *Buying the Wind: Regional Folklore in the United States.* Chicago and London: The University of Chicago Press, 1964.

Dougherty, Molly Crocker. "Southern Lay Midwives as Ritual Specialists." In *Women in Ritual and Symbolic Roles,* edited by Judith Hoch-Smith and Anita Spring, 151–164. New York: Plenum Press, 1978.

————. *Becoming a Woman in Rural Black Culture.* New York: Holt, Rinehart and Winston, 1978.

Dow, Thomas W. "Primitive Medicine in Haiti." *Bulletin of the History of Medicine* 39, 1 (1965): 34–52.

Droege, Thomas A. *The Faith Factor in Healing.* Philadelphia: Trinity Press International, 1991.

Duffy, John, ed. *History of Medicine in Louisiana.* 2 vols. Baton Rouge, La.: Louisiana State University, 1958.

Duke, James A. *CRC Handbook of Medicinal Herbs.* Boca Raton, Fla.: CRC Press, Inc., 1985.

Dunbar-Nelson, Alice. "People of Color in Louisiana, Part I." *Journal of Negro History* 1 (1916): 361–376.

————. "People of Color in Louisiana." *Journal of Negro History* 2 (1917): 67–69.

Dundes, Alan, ed. *Mother Wit from the Laughing Barrel: Readings in the Interpretation of Afro-American Folklore.* Englewood Cliffs, N.J.: Prentice-Hall, Inc., 1973.

————. *Analytic Essays in Folklore.* Edited by Richard M. Dorson. Paris: Mouton The Hague, 1975.

Dunham, Katherine. *Dances of Haiti.* Los Angeles: Center for Afro-American Studies/University of California, 1983.

Dupre, Gilbert. "Distinguished Opelousan Discourses on St. Landry." *Opelousas* (Louisiana) *Daily World,* June 12, 1970, 5.

Dye, Nancy Schrom. "History of Childbirth in America." *SIGNS: Journal of Women in Culture and Society* 6, 1 (1980): 97–108.

Eakin, Myrtle Sue. "The Black Struggle for Education in Louisiana, 1877–1930's." Ph.D. diss., University of Southwestern Louisiana, 1980.

Edwards, Jay. "Cultural Syncretism in the Louisiana Creole Cottage." *Louisiana Folklore Miscellany* 4 (1976–1980): 9–40.

Ehrenreich, Barbara, and Deirdre English. *For Her Own Good: 150 Years of the Experts' Advice to Women.* New York: Anchor Books, 1979.

Emery, Lynne Fauley. *Black Dance from 1619 to Today*. Princeton, N.J.: Princeton Book Company, 1988.

Evans-Pritchard, E. E. *Witchcraft, Oracles and Magic Among the Azande*. Oxford: Clarendon Press, 1937.

————. "The Morphology and Function of Magic: A Comparative Study of Trobriand and Zande Ritual and Spells." In *Magic, Witchcraft, and Curing*, edited by John Middleton, 1–22. Austin: University of Texas Press, 1967.

Everett, Thomas H. *The New York Botanical Garden Illustrated Encyclopedia of Horticulture*, vol. 9. New York and London: Garland Publishing, Inc., 1982.

Falanga, Gary. "Church Point Erases 'Coon Town,'" *Opelousas* (Louisiana) *Daily World*, August 3, 1989, 5a.

Fee, Elizabeth. "Women and Health Care: A Comparison of Theories," in *Seizing Our Bodies: The Politics of Women's Health*, edited by Claudia Dreifus, 279–297. New York: Vintage Books, 1977.

Felsher, John. "Spanish Moss: The Stuff of Legends." *Acadiana Profile: A Magazine About South Louisiana* 9 (1981): 14–38.

Fiehrer, Thomas Marc. "The African Presence in Colonial Louisiana: An Essay on the Continuity of Caribbean Culture." In *Louisiana's Black Heritage*, edited by Edward F. Haas, John R. Kemp, and Robert R. Macdonald, 3–31. New Orleans: Louisiana State Museum, 1979.

Fisher, Allyn. "The Bible Probed for Medical Clues." *Opelousas* (Louisiana) *Daily World*, January 26, 1988, 6.

Fitts, Leroy. *A History of Black Baptists*. Nashville, Tenn.: Broadman Press, 1985.

Fontenot, Marshall P. *Grand Prairie: Looking Back*. Opelousas, La.: Andrepont Printing Company, 1988.

Fontenot, Ruth Robertson. "An Opelousas History Beginning in 1690's." *Opelousas* (Louisiana) *Daily World*, June 12, 1970, 22–23.

Fontenot, Wonda L. "Madame Neau: The Practice of Ethno-psychiatry in Rural Louisiana." In *Wings of Gauze: Women of Color and the Experience of Health and Illness*, edited by Barbara Bair and Susan Cayleff, 41–52. Detroit: Wayne State University Press, 1993.

Ford, Richard I., ed. *The Nature and Status of Ethnobotany*, No. 67. Ann Arbor, Mich.: Museum of Anthropology, University of Michigan, 1978.

Fortier, Alcee. *A History of Louisiana, Volume 3, The American Domination 1803–1861*. New York: Manzi, Joyant and Company Successors, 1904.

Foster, George M., and Barbara Gallatin Anderson. *Medical Anthropology*. New York: John Wiley & Sons, 1978.

Frazer, Sir James George. *The Golden Bough: A Study in Magic and Religion*. 1922. Reprint. New York: The Macmillan Company, 1958.

Frazier, E. Franklin. *The Negro Church in America*. New York: Schocken Books, 1966.

Freeman, Harold, and Linda Villarosa. "Emergency: The Crisis in Our Health Care." *Essence* (September 1991): 59–62, 112–114.

Gahn, Robert Jr. *A History of Evangeline: Its Land, Its Men and Its Women Who Made it a Beautiful Place to Live*. Baton Rouge, La.: Claitor's Publishing Division, 1941.

Gaines, Atwood, D., ed. *Ethnopsychiatry: The Cultural Construction of Professional and Folk Psychiatries*. Albany: State University of New York Press, 1992.

Gardner, Gerald Brosseau. "British Charms, Amulets and Talismans." *Folk-Lore* 53 (1942): 95–103.

Garro, Linda Young. "The Ethnography of Health Care Decisions." *Social Science Medicine* 16 (1982): 1451–1452.

Gatschet, Albert S. *A Migration Legend of the Creek Indians: With a Linguistic, Historic and Ethnographic Introduction*, vol. 1. New York: AMS Press, 1884.

Germain, Carol P. "Cultural Care: A Bridge Between Sickness, Illness, and Disease." *Holistic Nursing Practice* 6, no. 3 (1992): 1–9.

Gilkes, Cheryl Townsend. "From Slavery to Social Welfare: Racism and the Control of Black Women." In *Class, Race, and Sex: The Dynamics of Control*, edited by Amy Swerdlow and Hanna Lessinger, 288–300. Boston: G. K. Hall and Company, 1983.

Glick, Leonard B. "Medicine as an Ethnographic Category: The Gimi of the New Guinea Highlands." *Ethnology* 6 (1967): 31–56.

Gonzalez, Marie, Victoria Barvera, Peter Guarnaccia, and Stephen L. Schensul. "'La Operacion': An Analysis of Sterilization in a Puerto Rican Community in Connecticut." In *Latina Women in Transition*, edited by R. E. Zambrana 47–62. Bronx, New York: Hispanic Research Center, Fordham University, 1982.

Gordon-Bradshaw, Ruth H. "A Social Essay on Special Issues Facing Poor Women of Color." *Women and Health* 12, nos. 3/4 (1987): 243–259.

Gould, Harold A. "The Implications of Technological Change for Folk and Scientific Medicine." *American Anthropologist* 59 (1957): 507–516.

Gray, Jim. Unpublished Papers, Sonoma State University, Sonoma, Cal., 1979.

Griffin, Amanda. "Today's Midwife is Noticeably Different." *Opelousas* (Louisiana) *Daily World*, October 4, 1987, 1c.

Griffin, Harry Lewis. *The Attakapa Country*. New Orleans: Pelican Publishing Company, 1959.

Grime, William, ed. *Botany of the Black Americans*. St. Clair Shores, Mich.: Scholarly Press, Inc., 1976.

Gunther, R. T. "The Cimaruta: Its Structure and Development." *Folk-Lore* 16 (1905): 133–155.

Gutman, Herbert G. "Marital and Sexual Norms Among Slave Women." In *A Heritage of Her Own: Toward a New Social History of American Women*, edited by Nancy F. Cott and Elizabeth H. Pleck, 298–310. New York: Simon and Schuster, 1979.

Hand, Wayland D. *The Frank Brown Collection of North Carolina Folklore: Popular Beliefs and Superstitions from North Carolina, Vols. 6 & 7*. Durham, N.C.: Duke University Press, 1964.

———. *Magical Medicine: The Folkloric Component of Medicine in Folk Belief, Custom, and Ritual of the Peoples of Europe and America*. Berkeley: University of California Press, 1980.

Handler, Jerome, and Frederick W. Lange. *Plantation Slavery in Barbados*. Cambridge, Mass.: Harvard University Press, 1978.

Handloff, Robert E. "Prayers, Amulets, and Charms: Health and Social Control." *African Studies Review* 25 (1982): 185–194.

Harley, George Way. *Native African Medicine: With Special Reference to its Practice in the Mano Tribe of Liberia*. 2d ed. London: Frank Cass and Co., Ltd., 1970.

Harvey, William M. "Black American Folk Healing." In *Folk Medicine and Herbal*

Healing, edited by George G. Meyer et. al., 153–165. Springfield, Ill.: Charles
C. Thomas Publishers, 1981.

Haskins, James. *Witchcraft, Mysticism and Magic in the Black World*. Garden City,
N.Y.: Doubleday & Company, Inc., 1974.

Herskovits, Melville J. *The Myth of the Negro Past*. Boston: Beacon Press, 1969.

Heyer, Kathryn W. "Some Psychological Implications of Changing Medical Practice
on the Sea Islands." In *Proceedings of a Symposium on Culture and Health:
Implications for Health Policy in Rural South Carolina*, edited by Melba S.
Varner, 50–65. Charleston, S.C.: College of Charleston, Center for Metropolitan
Affairs and Public Policy, 1979.

Hildburgh, Walter Leo. " 'Caravaca' Crosses and Their Uses as Amulets in Spain."
Folk-Lore 51 (1940): 241–58.

———. "Indeterminability and Confusion as Apotropaic Elements in Italy and in
Spain." *Folk-Lore* 55 (1944): 133–149.

———. "Psychology Underlying the Employment of Amulets." *Folk-Lore*, 62 (1951):
231–251.

Hill, Carole E. "Black Healing Practices in the Rural South." *Journal of Popular Culture*
6 (1973): 849–853.

———. "A Folk Medical Belief System in the American South: Some Practical Considerations." *Southern Medicine* 64 (1976): 11–17.

Hodges, David Julian. "The Cajun Culture of Southwestern Louisiana: A Study of
Cultural Isolation and Role Adaptation as Factors in the Fusion of Black African
and French Acadian Culture Traits." Ph.D. diss., New York University, 1972.

Holloway, Joseph E. *Africanisms in American Culture*. Bloomington: Indiana University
Press, 1990.

Holmes, Linda Janet. "Louvenia Taylor Benjamin, Southern Lay Midwife: An Interview." *SAGE* 2, no. 2 (1985): 51–54.

Honko, Lauri (Helsinki). "On the Effectivity of Folk Medicine." *Arv* 18–19 (1962–63):
290–300.

Howes, Michael. *Amulets*. New York: St. Martin Press, Inc., 1976.

Hudson, Charles M. *Four Centuries of Southern Indians*. Athens, Ga.: The University
of Georgia Press, 1975.

Hunt, Alfred N. *Haiti's Influence on Antebellum America: Slumbering Volcano in the
Caribbean*. Baton Rouge: Louisiana State University, 1988.

Hunter, K. I., M. W. Linn, and S. R. Stein. "Sterilization among American Indian and
Chicana Mothers," *International Quarterly of Community Health and Education*
4, no. 4 (1983–84): 343–352.

Hurston, Zora Neale. *Mules and Men: Negro Folktales and Voodoo Practices in the
South*. 1935. Reprint. New York: Harper and Row, Publishers, Inc., 1970.

———. *The Sanctified Church*. Berkeley: Turtle Island, 1983.

Hyatt, Harry Middleton. *Hoo-doo Conjuration-Witchcraft-Rootwork*. 6 vols. Cambridge, Md.: Memoirs of the Alma Egan Hyatt Foundation, 1973.

Hymes, Dell, ed. *Pidginization and Creolization of Languages*. London: Cambridge
University Press, 1971.

Idowu, E. Bolaji. *Olodumare: God in Yoruba Belief*. London: Longmans, 1962.

Imperato, Pascal James. *African Folk Medicine: Practices and Beliefs of the Bambara
and Other Peoples*. Baltimore: York Press, Inc., 1977.

Jackson, Bruce. "The Other Kind of Doctor: Conjure and Magic in Black American

Folk Medicine." In *American Folk Medicine: A Symposium*, edited by Wayland D. Hand, 259–272. Berkeley: University of California Press, 1980.

Jaco, E. Gartly, ed. *Patients, Physicians, and Illness: A Sourcebook in Behavioral Science and Health*. New York: The Free Press, 1979.

Jenkins, Velesta. "River Road: A Rural Black Community in Southeastern Louisiana." Ph.D. diss., University of California, Berkeley, 1976.

Johnston, Maxene. "Folk Beliefs and Ethnocultural Behavior in Pediatrics." *Nursing Clinics of North America* 12, 1 (1977): 77–87.

Jones, David. E. *Sanapia: Comanche Medicine Woman*. Prospect Heights, Ill.: Waveland Press, 1972.

Jones, Joseph Hardy, Jr. "The People of Frilot Cove: A Study of a Racial Hybrid Community in Rural South Central Louisiana." M. A. thesis, Louisiana State University, 1950.

Jones, Wilken, Jr. *The Beginning of Something Good: Plaisance High School*. Plaisance, La.: Author, 1980.

Jones-Jackson, Patricia. *When Roots Die: Endangered Traditions on the Sea Islands*. Athens and London: The University of Georgia Press, 1987.

Jordan, Rosan A., and Susan J. Kalcik, eds. *Women's Folklore, Women's Culture*. Philadelphia: University of Pennsylvania Press, 1985.

Jordan, Weymouth T. "Plantation Medicine in the Old South." *The Alabama Review* 3, no. 2 (1950): 83–107.

Joyner, Charles. *Down by the Riverside: A South Carolina Slave Community*. Urbana and Chicago: University of Illinois Press, 1984.

Katz, William Loren. *Black Indians: A Hidden Heritage*. New York: Atheneum/Macmillan Publishing Company, 1986.

Kendall, John Smith. "The Huntsmen of Black Ivory." *The Louisiana Historical Quarterly* 24 (1941): 9–34.

Kiev, Ari., ed. *Magic, Faith, and Healing: Studies in Primitive Psychiatry Today*. New York: The Free Press, 1964.

King, Mike. "Blacks are Penalized by Tier System Says Study." *Opelousas* (Louisiana) *Daily World*, February 9, 1990, 2a.

Kirkham, Mavis. "A Feminist Perspective in Midwifery." In *Feminist Practice in Women's Health Care*, edited by Christine Webb, 35–49. New York: John Wiley & Sons, 1986.

Kniffen, Fred B. "The Historic Indian Tribes of Louisiana," *Louisiana Conservation Review* 4 (1935): 5–12.

Kniffen, Fred B., Hiram F. Gregory, and George A. Stokes. *The Historic Indian Tribes of Louisiana: From 1542 to the Present*. Baton Rouge and London: Louisiana State University, 1987.

Krochmal, Connie, and Arnold Krochmal. *A Field Guide to Medicinal Plants*. New York: Times Books, 1973.

Kuna, Ralph R. "Hoodoo: The Indigenous Medicine and Psychiatry of the Black America." *EthnoMedicine* 3 (1974/75): 273–294.

Ladner, Joyce A. "Racism and Tradition: Black Womanhood in Historical Perspective." In *Liberating Women's History: Theoretical and Critical Essays*, edited by Bernice A. Carroll, 179–193. Chicago: University of Illinois Press, 1976.

LaFargue, Andre. "The Louisiana Purchase: The French Viewpoint." *The Louisiana Historical Quarterly* 23 (1940): 107–117.

Laguerre, Michel. *Afro-Caribbean Folk Medicine*. South Hadley, Mass.: Bergin & Garvey Publishers, Inc., 1987.

Lancon, John Adrain. "Des Remedes aux Traiteurs: An Introduction to Folk Medicine in French Louisiana." Lafayette, La.: University of Southwestern Louisiana, 1986.

Landry, Garrie. "Some of the Medicinal Plants that Figured in the Domestic Practices of Lafayette Parish." Unpublished papers, University of Southwestern Louisiana, Lafayette, 1989.

Lange, Yvonne. "Lithography, an Agent of Technological Change in Religion Folk Art: A Thesis." *Western Folklore* 33 (1974): 51–64.

Langley, Sarah, and B. Berthold Wolff. "Cultural Factors and the Response to Pain: A Review." *American Anthropologist* 70 (1968): 494–501.

Lawhorne, L., et al. "Children and Pregnant Women." *Journal of Rural Health* 6, 4 (1990): 365–377.

Leonard, Roscoe, and Clude Oubre. "Free and Proud: St. Landry's Gens de Couleur." In *Louisiana Tapestry: The Ethnic Weave of St. Landry Parish*, edited by Vaughan B. Baker and Jean T. Kreamer, 70–81. Lafayette, La.: Center for Louisiana Studies, University of Southwestern Louisiana, 1983.

Levine, Lawrence. *Black Culture and Black Consciousness: Afro-American Folk Thought from Slavery to Freedom*. London: Oxford University Press, 1977.

Lewin, Ellen, and Virginia Olesen, eds. *Women, Health and Healing: Toward a New Perspective*. New York: Tavistock Publications, 1985.

Lex, Barbara W. "Voodoo Death: New Thoughts on an Old Explanation." *American Anthropologist* 76 (1974): 818–823.

Long, Charles H. *Significations: Signs, Symbols, and Images in the Interpretation of Religion*. Philadelphia: Fortress Press, 1986.

Long, Jim. "Patent Medicines," *The Herb Companion* 5 (1993): 48–52.

Lopez, Iris. "Sterilization Among Puerto Rican Women in New York City: Public Policy and Social Constraints." In *Cities of the United States: Studies in Urban Anthropology*, edited by Leith Mullings. New York: Columbia University Press, 1987.

Malveaux, Julianne, and Margaret C. Simms, eds. *Slipping Through the Cracks: The Statue of Black Women*. New Brunswick, N.J.: Transaction Publishers, 1989.

Marc De Villiers du Terrage. *The Last Years of French Louisiana*. Translated by Hosea Phillips. Edited by Carl A. Brasseaux and Glenn R. Conrad. Lafayette, La.: Center for Louisiana Studies, University of Southwestern Louisiana, 1982.

Marieskind, Helen. "The Women's Health Movement." *International Journal of Health Services Research* 5, 2 (1975): 217–223.

Martin, Thad. "The Disappearing Black Farmer." *Ebony* (June 1985): 145–151.

May, Herbert J., Jr. "The Official Policy of the Roman Catholic Church of the Diocese of Lafayette in Relation to Black Catholics, 1940 to 1978." M. A. Thesis, University of Southwestern Louisiana, 1981.

Mbiti, John S. *African Religions and Philosophy*. Garden City, N.Y.: Anchor Books/Doubleday and Company, Inc., 1970.

McClain, Carol Shepherd, ed. *Women as Healers: Cross-Cultural Perspectives*. New Brunswick, N.J. and London: Rutgers University Press, 1989.

McIntyre, Charshee C. L. *Criminalizing a Race: Free Blacks During Slavery*. Queens, N.Y.: Kayode Publications, Ltd., 1993.

McMurtrie, Douglas C. "A Louisiana Decree of 1770 Relative to the Practice of Medicine and Surgery." *New Orleans Medical and Surgical Journal* 86 (1933): 7–11.

Mellette, Ramsey. "Culture-Bound Syndrome: Concerns of a Psychiatrist." In *Proceedings of a Symposium on Culture and Health: Implications for Health Policy in Rural South Carolina*, edited by Melba S. Varner, 79–85. Charleston, S.C.: College of Charleston, Center for Metropolitan Affairs and Public Policy, 1979.

Melville, Margarita B., ed. *Twice a Minority: Mexican American Women*. St. Louis, Toronto, and London: The C. V. Mosby Company, 1980.

Messer, Ellen. "Present and Future Prospects of Herbal Medicine in a Mexican Community." In *The Nature and Status of Ethnobotany*, edited by Richard I. Ford, 137–160. Ann Arbor, Mich.: Museum of Anthropology, University of Michigan, 1978.

Metcalf, Peter. *Where Are You Spirits: Style and Theme in Berawan Prayer*. Washington, D.C.: Smithsonian Institution Press, 1989.

Metraux, Alfred. *Voodoo in Haiti*. Translated by Hugo Charteris. New York: Schocken Books, 1972.

Middleton, John, and E. H. Winter, eds. *Witchcraft and Sorcery in West Africa*. New York: Frederick A. Praeger, 1963.

Miller, Kelly. "The Historic Background of the Negro Physician." *The Journal of Negro History* 1 (1916): 99–109.

Mintz, Sidney, and Richard Price. *An Anthropological Approach to the African American Past: A Caribbean Perspective*. Philadelphia: Institute for the Study of Human Issues, 1976.

Mitchell, Ella P. "Oral Tradition: Legacy of Faith for the Black Church." *Religious Education* 81 (1986): 93–112.

Mitchell, Faith. *Hoodoo Medicine: Sea Islands Herbal Medicines*. San Francisco, Calif.: Reed, Cannon & Johnson Co., 1978.

Mitchell, Henry. *Black Belief: Folk Beliefs of Blacks in America and West Africa*. New York: Harper & Row, Publishers, 1975.

Moore, Kathryn. "Seed Jewelry: Seeds Used as Beads—Facts and Folklore." *Plant Lore* 6 (1982): 19–27.

Morais, Herbert M. *The History of the Negro in Medicine*. New York, Washington, and London: International Library of Negro Life and History, Publisher's Company, Inc., 1967.

Morazan, Ronald R. "Some Spanish Contributions to the Uniqueness of Louisiana." In *Louisiana Tapestry: The Ethnic Weave of St. Landry Parish*, edited by Vaughan B. Baker and Jean T. Kreamer, 91–97. Lafayette, La.: Center for Louisiana Studies, University of Southwestern Louisiana, 1983.

Morgan, Sandra, ed. *Gender and Anthropology: Critical Reviews for Research and Teaching*. Washington, D.C.: American Anthropological Association, 1989.

Morton, Julia F. *Atlas of Medicinal Plants of Middle America: Bahamas to Yucatan*. Springfield, Ill.: Charles Thomas Publisher, 1981.

Mullings, Leith. *Therapy, Ideology, and Social Change: Mental Health Healing in Urban Ghana*. Berkeley: University of California Press, 1984.

———. ed. *Cities of the United States: Studies in Urban Anthropology*. New York: Columbia University Press, 1987.

Murphree, Alice. "Plants in Florida Folk Medicine." *Florida Anthropologist* 18 (1965): 175–185.

————. "Folk Beliefs; Understanding of Health, Illness, and Treatment." In *The Health of a Rural County: Perspectives and Problems*, edited by Richard C. Reynolds, Sam A. Banks, and Alice Murphree, 111–123. Gainesville, Fl.: The University Presses of Florida, 1976.

Myers, Cheryl Bihm. *Palmetto: The Early Years*. Opelousas, La.: Bodemuller the Printer, Inc., 1987.

Nassau, Rev. Robert Hamill. *Fetichism in West Africa: Forty Years' Observation of Native Customs and Superstitions*. London: Duckworth & Co., 1904.

Newton, Lewis William. "The Americanization of French Louisiana: A Study of the Process of Adjustment Between the French and the Anglo American Populations of Louisiana, 1803–1860." Ph.D. diss., University of Chicago, 1929.

Niethammer, Carolyn. *Daughters of the Earth: The Lives and Legends of American Indian Women*. New York: Macmillan Publishing Co., Inc., 1977.

Normand, Keith. "Farming Remains Parish's Largest Industry." *Daily World*, August 14, 1989, 9.

Oduyoye, Modupe. *The Vocabulary of Yoruba Religious Discourse*. Ibadan, Nigeria: Daystar Press, 1971.

O'Joade, J. Olowo. "The Nigerian Folklore of Faith-Healing: The example of a Jos-based Nigerian Faith Healer." Unpublished manuscript, Centre for Development Studies, University of Jos, Jos, Nigeria, 1986.

O'Keefe, Lawrence Daniel. *Stolen Lighting: The Social Theory of Magic*. New York: The Continuum Publishing Company, 1982.

Olsen, Virginia, and Ellen Lewin. "Women, Health, and Healing: A Theoretical Introduction." In *Women, Health, and Healing: Toward a New Perspective*, edited by Virginia Olsen and Ellen Lewin. New York: Tavistock Publications, 1985.

Oubre, Claude F. "The Freedmen's Bureau and Negro Land Ownership." M. A. Thesis, University of Southwestern Louisiana, 1970.

————. "The Opelousas Riot of 1868." *Attakapas Gazette* 7 (1973): 139–152.

Paredes, J. Anthony. "The Folk Culture of the Eastern Creek Indians: Synthesis and Change." In *A Creek Sourcebook*, edited by William C. Sturtevant, 93–111. New York: Garland Publishing, Inc.

Peterson, John H., Jr. "Louisiana Choctaw Life at the End of the Nineteenth Century." In *Four Centuries of Southern Indians*, edited by Charles Hudson. Athens, Ga.: The University of Georgia Press, 1975.

Petterson, Olof. "Magic and Medicine in South African Bantu Psychiatry." *Centaurus* 9 (1963): 293–316.

Piersen, William D. *Black Yankees: The Development of an Afro-American Subculture in Eighteenth Century New England*. Amherst, Mass.: The University of Massachusetts Press, 1988.

Pinkney, Alphonso. *Black Americans*. 4th ed. Englewood Cliffs, N.J.: Prentice Hall, 1993.

Pipes, William H. *Say Amen, Brother! Old Time Negro Preaching: A Study in American Frustration*. Westport, Conn.: Negro Universities Press, 1970 [1951].

Pitts, Walter F. *Old Ship of Zion: The Afro-Baptist Ritual in the African Diaspora*. New York: Oxford University Press, 1993.

Poloma, Margaret M., and George H. Gallup, Jr. *Varieties of Prayer: A Survey Report*. Philadelphia: Trinity Press International, 1991.

Porcher, Francis Peyre. *Southern Fields and Forests: Medical, Economical and Agri-*

cultural. Being Also a Medical Botany of the Confederate States. Charleston, S.C.: Steam Power Press of Evans and Cogswell, 1863.

Porteous, Laura L. "The Gri Gri Case, A Criminal Trial in Louisiana During the Spanish Regime, 1773." *The Louisiana Historical Quarterly* 17 (1934): 48–63.

Post, Lauren C. "Some Notes on the Attakapas Indians of Southwest Louisiana." *Louisiana History* 3 (1962): 221–243.

Postell, William Dosite. *The Health of Slaves on Southern Plantations.* Baton Rouge: Louisiana State University Press, 1951.

Potter, Kenneth. "Relations Between Negroes and Indians Within the Present Limits of the United States." *Journal of Negro History* 17 (1932): 287–367.

———. "Relations Between Negroes and Indians Within the Present Limits of the United States." *Journal of Negro History* 18 (1933): 282–321.

Prince, Raymond. "Indigenous Yoruba Psychiatry." In *Magic, Faith, and Healing: Studies in Primitive Psychiatry Today*, edited by Ari Kiev, 84–120. New York: The Free Press, 1964.

Puckett, Newbell Niles. *Folk Beliefs of the Southern Negro.* New York: Negro Universities Press, 1926.

Raboteau, Albert J. *Slave Religion: The "Invisible Institution" in the Antebellum South.* Oxford: Oxford University Press, 1980.

Rawick, George P., ed. *The American Slave: A Composite Autobiography, From Sundown to Sunup: The Making of the Black Community*, vol. 1. Westport, Conn.: Greenwood Publishing Company, 1972.

———., ed. *The American Slave: A Composite Autobiography, God Struck Me Dead*, vol. 19. Westport, Conn.: Greenwood Publishing Company, 1972.

Richardson, Hilda. "The Health Plight of Rural Women." *Women and Health* 12, 3/4, (1987): 41–54.

Rickels, Patricia K. "The Folklore of Acadiana." In *The Culture of Acadiana: Tradition and Change in South Louisiana*, edited by Steven L. Del Sesto and Jon L. Gibson, 143–174. Lafayette: The Center for Louisiana Studies, University of Southwestern Louisiana, 1975.

Rickford, John R. "The Question of Prior Creolization in Black English." In *Pidgin and Creole Linguistics*, edited by Albert Valdman, 190–221. Bloomington: Indiana University Press, 1977.

Rivers, W.H.R. *Medicine, Magic, and Religion: The Fitz Patrick Lectures delivered before the Royal College of Physicians of London in 1915 and 1916.* New York: Harcourt, Brace and Company, Inc., 1924.

Robbins, Wilfred William, John Peabody Harrington, and Barbara Freire-Marreco. *Ethnobotany of the Tewa Indians.* Washington, D.C.: Bureau of American Ethnology, Bulletin 55, Government Printing Office, 1916.

Roberts, Hilda. "Louisiana Superstitions." *Journal of American Folklore* 40 (1927): 144–208.

Robertson, James Alexander, ed. *Louisiana: Under the Rule of Spain, France, and the United States 1785–1807.* 1910. Reprint. Freeport, N.Y.: Books for Libraries Press, 1969.

Robin, C. C. *Voyage to Louisiana, 1803–1805.* Translated by Stuart O. Landry. New Orleans: Pelican Publishing, Co., 1966.

Robinson, Jean. "Black Healers During the Colonial Period and Early 19th Century America." Ph.D. diss., Southern Illinois University, 1979.

Rogler, Lloyd H., and August B. Hollingshead. "The Puerto Rican Spiritualist As A Psychiatrist." *The American Journal of Sociology* 67, 1 (1961): 17–21.

Roheim, Geza. *Animism, Magic and the Divine King*. New York: Alfred A. Knopf, 1930.

Rousseve, Charles Barthelemy. *The Negro in Louisiana: Aspects of his History and his Literature*. New Orleans: The Xavier University Press, 1937.

Sanders, Albert Godfrey. "Documents Covering the Beginning of the African Slave Trade in Louisiana, 1718." *The Louisiana Historical Quarterly* 14 (1931): 172–177.

Satariano, William A., Steven H. Belle, and G. Marie Swanson. "The Severity of Breast Cancer at Diagnosis: A Comparison of Age and Extent of Disease in Black and White Women." *American Journal of Public Health* 76, 7 (1986): 779–782.

Savitt, Todd L. *Medicine and Slavery: The Diseases and Health Care of Blacks in Antebellum Virginia*. Urbana, Chicago, and London: University of Illinois Press, 1978.

Schaffer, Ruth C. "The Health and Social Functions of Black Midwives on the Texas Brazos Bottom, 1920–1985." *Rural Sociology* 56, no. 1 (1991): 89–105.

Schneider, Jane, and Annette B. Weiner, eds. *Cloth and Human Experience*. Washington and London: Smithsonian Institution Press, 1989.

Seale, Lee, and Marianna Seale. "Easter Rock: A Louisiana Negro Ceremony." *Journal of American Folklore* 55 (1942): 212–217.

Seijas, Haydee. "An Approach to the Study of the Medical Aspects of Culture." *Current Anthropology* 14 (1973): 544–545.

Sewell, S. S. "Sterilization Abuse and Hispanic Women." In *Birth Control and Controlling Birth*, edited by H. B. Holmes, B. B. Hoskines, and M. Gross, 121–124. Clifton, N.Y.: Humana Press, 1980.

Shapiro, T. *Population Control Politics: Women, Sterilization, and Reproductive Choice*. Philadelphia: Temple University Press, 1985.

Shorter, Aylward. *Prayer in the Religious Traditions of Africa*. New York: Oxford University Press, 1975.

Simmons, William S. *Eyes of the Night: Witchcraft Among a Senegalese People*. Boston: Little, Brown and Company, 1971.

———. *Spirit of the New England Tribes: Indian History and Folklore, 1620–1984*. Hanover, N.H. and London: University of New England, 1986.

Simpson, George Eaton. *Black Religions in the New World*. New York: Columbia University Press, 1978.

Singleton, Theresa A. "The Archaeology of African American Life." *Anthro News* 12 (1990): 1–4, 14.

Smith, J. Alfred. "The Role of the Black Clergy as Allied Health Care Professionals in Working with Black Patients." In *Black Awareness: Implications for Black Patient Care*, edited by Dorothy Luckraft. New York: The American Journal of Nursing Co., 1976.

Smitherman, Geneva. *Talking and Testifying: The Language of Black America*. Detroit: Wayne State University Press, 1977.

Snow, Loudell F. "The Religious Component in Southern Folk Medicine." In *Traditional Healing: New Science or New Colonialism? (Essays in Critique of Medical Anthropology)*, edited by Philip Singer, 26–51. New York and London: Conch Magazine, Ltd., 1977a.

———. "Popular Medicine in a Black Neighborhood." In *Ethnic Medicine in the South-*

west, edited by Edward H. Spicer, 19–95. Tucson: The University of Arizona Press, 1977b.

―――. "I Was Born Just Exactly With the Gift: An Interview With a Voodoo Practitioner." *Journal of American Folklore* 99 (1986): 272–281.

Sobel, Mechal. *Trabelin' On: The Slave Journey to an Afro-Baptist Faith.* Westport, Conn. and London: Greenwood Press, 1979.

Sofowora, Abayomi. *Medicinal Plants and Traditional Medicine in Africa.* Chichester, N.Y.: John Wiley and Sons, Ltd., 1982.

Sojourner, Sabrina. "From the House of Yemanja: The Goddess Heritage of Black Women." In *The Politics of Women's Spirituality*, edited by Charlene Spretnak, 57–63. New York: Anchor/Doubleday, 1982.

Souchon, Edmond. *Original Contributions of Louisiana to Medical Sciences: A Biographic Study.* New Orleans: American Pig Co., 1915.

Southern, Eileen. *The Music of Black Americans: A History.* 2d ed. New York: W. W. Norton & Company, 1971.

Spencer, Debra. "Is Racism Killing Us?" *Essence* (January 1993): 31–34.

Spring, Anita, and Judith Hoch-Smith. *Women in Ritual and Symbolic Roles.* New York: Plenum Press, 1978.

Stampp, Kenneth M. *The Peculiar Institution: Slavery in the Ante-Bellum South.* New York: Vintage Press, 1956.

Sterkx, H. E. *The Free Negro in Ante-Bellum Louisiana.* Rutherford, N.J.: Fairleigh Dickinson University Press, 1972.

Stewart, Horace. "Kindling of Hope in the Disadvantage: A Study of the Afro-American Healer." *Mental Hygiene* 55 (1971): 96–100.

Stuart, Eileen M., John P. Deckro, and Carol Lynn Mandle. "Spirituality in Health and Healing: A Clinical Program." *Holistic Nursing Practice* 3, 3 (1989): 35–36.

Sturtevant, William C. "Seminole Myths on The Origins of Races." *Ethnohistory* 10 (1963): 80–86.

Sutton, Joelbrett. "Spirit and Polity in a Black Primitive Baptist Church." Ph.D. diss., University of North Carolina at Chapel Hill, 1983.

Swanton, John R. *Indian Tribes of the Lower Mississippi Valley and Adjacent Coast of the Gulf of Mexico.* Washington, D.C.: Bureau of American Ethnology, Bulletin 43, Government Printing Office, 1911.

―――. *A Structural and Lexical Comparison of the Tunica, Chitimacha, and Atakapa Languages.* Washington, D.C.: Bureau of Ethnology, Bulletin 68, Government Printing Office, 1919.

―――. *Early History of the Creek Indians and Their Neighbors.* Washington, D.C.: Bureau of American Ethnology, Bulletin 73, Government Printing Office, 1922.

―――. *The Indians of the Southeastern United States.* Washington, D.C.: Bureau of American Ethnology, Bulletin 137, Government Printing Office, 1946.

Tallant, Robert. *Voodoo: In New Orleans.* New York: Collier Books, 1967.

Taylor, David D., and Dale R. Thomas. *Contributions of the Herbarium of Northeast Louisiana University*, No. 6. Monroe, La.: The Herbarium, Northeast Louisiana University, 1985.

Taylor, Gertrude. "Early History of the Chitimacha," *Attakapas Gazette* 19 (1979): 65–69.

Taylor, Joe Gray. *Negro Slavery in Louisiana.* Baton Rouge: Louisiana Historical Society, Louisiana State University Press, 1963.

Tentchoff, Dorice. "Cajun French and French Creole: Their Speakers and the Question of Identities." In *The Culture of Acadiana: Tradition and Change in South Louisiana,* edited by Steven L. DelSesto and Jon L. Gibson, 87–107. Lafayette, La.: Center for Louisiana Studies, University of Southwestern Louisiana, 1975.

Thistlethwaite, John. "Opelousas-St. Landry Historic Summary." *Daily World,* June 12, 1970, 33–36.

Thompson, Robert Ferris. *The Flash of the Spirit: African & Afro-American Art & Philosophy.* New York: Vintage Books, 1984.

Ti'erou, Alphonse. *Doople': The Eternal Law of African Dance.* Philadelphia: Harwood Academic Publishers, 1992.

Tinling, David C. "Voodoo, Rootwork, and Medicine," *Psychosomatic Medicine: Journal of the American Psychosomatic Society* 29, no. 5 (1967): 483–490.

Touchstone, Samuel J. *Herbal and Folk Medicine of Louisiana and Adjacent States.* Princeton, La.: Folk-Life Books, 1983.

Turner, Victor. *Dramas, Fields, and Metaphors: Symbolic Action in Human Society.* Ithaca: Cornell University Press, 1974.

Tylor, Edward B. *Primitive Culture: Researches into the Development of Mythology, Philosophy, Religion, Language, Art, and Custom,* vols. 1 and 2. London: John Murray, Albemarle Street, W., 1920.

Underwood, Jane H. *Bicultural Interactions and Human Variation.* Dubuque, Iowa: Wm. C. Brown, 1975.

Usner, Daniel H., Jr. "From African Captivity to American Slavery: The Introduction of Black Laborers to Colonial Louisiana." *Louisiana History* 20 (1979): 25–48.

Valdman, Albert, ed. *Pidgin and Creole Linguistics.* Bloomington: Indiana University Press, 1977.

———. "Creolization and Second Language Acquisition." In *Pidginization and Creolization: As Language Acquisition,* edited by Roger W. Andersen, 212–234. Los Angeles: University of California Press, 1983.

Vansina, Jan. *Oral Tradition as History.* Madison, Wis.: The University of Wisconsin Press, 1985.

Verbrugge, Lois M., and Richard P. Steiner. "Physician Treatment of Men and Women Patients: Sex Bias or Appropriate Care?" *Medical Care* 19, 6 (1981): 609–632.

Vlach, John Michael. *The Afro-American Tradition in Decorative Art.* Cleveland, Ohio: The Cleveland Museum of Art, 1978.

Vogel, Virgil. "American Indian Influence on the American Pharmacopeia." In *Folk Medicine and Herbal Healing,* edited by George G. Meyer et al., 103–113. Springfield, Ill.: Charles C. Thomas Publisher, 1981.

Walker, Sheila S. "African Gods in the Americas: The Black Religious Continuum." *The Black Scholar* (1980): 25–36.

Washington, Joseph R., Jr. *Black Religion: The Negro and Christianity in the United States.* Boston: Beacon Press, 1964.

Watson, Wilbur H., ed. *Black Folk Medicine: The Therapeutic Significance of Faith and Trust.* New Brunswick, N.J.: Transaction Books, 1984.

Wattleton, Faye. "Teenage Pregnancy: A Case for National Action." In *The Black Women's Health Book: Speaking for Ourselves,* edited by Evelyn C. White, 107–111. Seattle: The Seal Press, 1990.

Webb, Julie Yvonne. "Louisiana Voodoo and Superstitions Related to Health." *HSMHA Health Reports* 86 (1971): 291–301.

Weiss, Kenneth R. "Push to Lower Infant Death Rate Begins." *Opelousas* (Louisiana) *Daily World*, February 9, 1990, 2a.

Wenger, Mark J. *A History of Washington Louisiana*. Lafayette: The Center for Louisiana Studies, University of Southwestern Louisiana, 1974.

West, Martin. *Bishops and Prophets in a Black City: African Independent Churches in Soweto Johannesburg*. London: David Philip, Publisher, 1975.

White, Evelyn C., ed. *The Black Women's Health Book: Speaking for Ourselves*. Seattle: Seal Press, 1990.

Whitten, Norman E. Jr. "Contemporary Patterns of Malign Occultism Among Negroes in North Carolina." In *Mother Wit from the Laughing Barrel: Readings in the Interpretation of Afro-American Folklore*, edited by Alan Dundes, 402–418. Englewood Cliffs, N.J.: Prentice-Hall, Inc. 1973.

Wilkerson, Margaret B., and Jewell Handy Gresham. "The Racialization of Poverty." *The Nation* 249, no. 4 (1989): 126–131.

Williams, Richard Allen. "Black Related Diseases: An Overview." *Journal of Black Health Perspective* 1 (1974): 35–40.

Wimbs, Cassandra "African-American Theory, Beliefs, and Practices: Candle Shops." M. A. Thesis, University of California, Berkeley, 1989.

Wingate, J. S. (Mrs.) "The Scroll of Cyprian: An Armenian Family Amulet." *Folklore* 41 (1930): 169–187.

Winston, Diane. "*More Americans Turn to Prayer Over Problems*." *Opelousas* (Louisiana) *Daily World*, March 25, 1990, 1, back page.

Wright, Leitch, Jr. *The Only Land They Knew: The Tragic Story of the American Indians in the Old South*. New York: The Free Press, 1981.

Zambrana, Ruth. "A Research Agenda on Issues Affecting Poor and Minority Women: A Model for Understanding Their Health Needs." *Women and Health* 12, nos. 3/4 (1987): 137–160.

Zeidenstein, Sondra, ed. "Learning About Rural Women." *Studies in Family Planning* 10, nos. 11/12 (November/December 1979): 309–314.

Index

African House, 12
Alabamas, 6, 9
Amulets: Biblical scroll, 116-17; color symbolism, 121–22, 126; compound, 116; cross symbolism, 121; definition of, 118; enumeration symbolism, 123–24, 126; fees for, 118-19; inscriptions on, 122–23; multi-knot string, 115; prayer bead necklace, 115; prayer cloth, 115–16; religious lithography, 74, 117–18; root necklace, 115; silver coin, 118; single-knot string, 114–15; social conflict and, 125–26; structure and function of, 118-21; walking cane, 117
Ardra, color red in, 122
Atakapas, 4, 6, 8
Avery, Bylly, 93

Bambara, 12, 115, 117
Baptists, 19
Beedeau, secret doctor, 63–64, 122, 123
Biblical scroll amulet, 116–17
Black Codes, 13–14

Bondoukou, Ivory Coast, 122–23
Bowman, Elisha, 10

Cajuns in Opelousas Territory, 11
Call and response prayer, 103–4
Caravaca cross, 121
Catholic churches, separate black and white, 20–21
Catholicism, introduction of, 13, 19
Catnip tea, 129
Cesarean section, 32
Cherokees, 123
Childhood diseases, 68-69
Chitimacha, 6, 8
Choctaws, 6, 9; Bayou Lacomb, 132
Christian, Barbara, 85–86
Christianity, Africanization of, 121, 134–35
Church schools, 21
Clarke, Adele, 96–97
Codes Noir, 13–14
Color symbolism, 121–22, 126
Compound amulet, 116
Conversational prayer, 101
Corn, use of, 128, 129
Cornmeal, use of, 125, 129

About the Author

WONDA FONTENOT is Executive Director of Wannamuse Institute for the Study of Arts, Culture, and Ethnicity in Opelousas, Louisiana. She is also a consultant in health care and rural African-American traditions. She has published a study of "Madame Neau: The Practice of Ethno-Psychiatry in Rural Louisiana" in *Wings of Gauze: Women of Color and the Experience of Health and Illness* (1993).

ISBN 0-89789-354-9

HARDCOVER BAR CODE